Pra... ...Dr. Charlotte... ...and
The... ...nation

"Simple, practica... ...l it will be when all
families give thei... ...r. Reznick's book.
Joy, success . . . and health and happiness are just around the corner!"
—Harvey Karp, MD, FAAP, creator of the book and
DVD *The Happiest Toddler on the Block*

"Dr. Reznick offers a revolutionary approach for parents to help their children handle fears, worries, and self-doubt. Her simple, accessible advice allows kids to develop their self-esteem while creatively tackling problems. This book is a must-read for any parent who hopes to arm their child with the tools to handle life's daily struggles."
—Jack Canfield, coauthor of *The Success Principles* and
coauthor of the Chicken Soup for the Soul series

"This is a wonderful guide for anyone raising children in a stressful world. I'm looking forward to practicing Dr. Reznick's strategies with my own daughters as they grow and become more aware of life's everyday pressures."
—Mallika Chopra, coauthor of *100 Questions from My Child*
and author of *100 Promises to My Baby*

"'The way out is through the inside.' This is how this profound guide for joy and success begins . . . right where it should. Charlotte knows kids, and she also knows the power of our own minds to heal ourselves, create images of joy, and become the things we believe we are. Join Charlotte in this journey into a very practical tool set for this age . . . helping our children to cope with all that is around them. It couldn't have come at a better time!"   —Lee Carroll, coauthor of the Indigo Children series

"As a skilled psychologist, Dr. Reznick draws from her wealth of experience to offer children and parents a treasure trove of skills to relieve stress. She presents well-written, easy-to-follow tools to use in every situation. From visualization techniques to breathing exercises, Dr. Reznick taps the power of a child's imagination to ensure kids achieve peace and success."
—Judith Orloff, MD, author of *Emotional Freedom*

continued . . .

"Charlotte Reznick shows how kids can access the power of their imaginations for healing, growth, learning, change, and peak performance. Her practical wisdom and considerable experience provide the groundwork and the actual imagery tools to reach all kinds of kids—rich and poor, smart kids and learning disabled, confident and unsure—not to mention their parents, teachers, and counselors. This is a wonderful resource!"

—Belleruth Naparstek, LISW, author of *Invisible Heroes* and creator of the Health Journeys audio series

"This is one of the most important books ever written because it teaches you how to teach your kids to deal with fear, anger, anxiety, illnesses, losses, and relationships in positive and healthy ways. Imagination is what makes humans different from all other creatures, yet nobody ever teaches us how to use it. Dr. Reznick, who has taught thousands of kids to use their imaginations for health and wellness, shows you how to teach your kids to use their mind/body connection to relax, sleep, study, heal, and have healthy responses to life's emotional challenges. *Every* parent, educator, and health-care worker should read this book."

—Martin L. Rossman, MD, author of *Guided Imagery for Self-Healing*

"*The Power of Your Child's Imagination* is one of the best creative books for children that I have read. Dr. Reznick clearly 'gets' children and understands their fears. In this book she provides the tools for children to empower themselves to climb out of fear, stress, and pain through their own imagination. This book can guide parents in how to help their children feel good about themselves and competent in the face of stressful situations and internal fears. This book is a must for all families with children."

—Lonnie Zeltzer, MD, director of the Pediatric Pain Program at Mattel Children's Hospital UCLA

"Charlotte Reznick's book is well written and eminently usable. It fills a gap that has existed for far too long. Imagery is a powerful tool for healing at all ages, and children have the greatest ability to utilize it. Every helping professional and every parent needs to learn these skills. I know of no better way to learn them than through this fine work."

—Emmett Miller, MD, author of *Deep Healing* and *Our Culture on the Couch*

"Charlotte Reznick has been a gift to so many of my patients, providing children and their families with a unique set of skills to address stress and solve issues. Now this toolbox is available to everyone. Parents will thank her for this inventive way of helping their children."

—Cara Natterson, MD, author of *Dangerous or Safe?*
Which Foods, Medicines, and Chemicals Really Put Your Kids at Risk

"*The Power of Your Child's Imagination* is a treasure chest of imagery-based interventions that can help parents deal more effectively with common childhood challenges. As Dr. Reznick advocates, teaching children to utilize the power of their imagination gives them critical tools for achieving success in all that they do. Every parent should familiarize themselves with the information contained in this book."

—David E. Bresler, PhD, LAc, president of the Academy for
Guided Imagery and founder and former executive director
of the UCLA Pain Control Unit

"The power of our imaginations to quickly and dramatically change our lives is profound. Charlotte Reznick makes this process clear, easy, and magical for children and the adults who love them."

—Mimi Doe, founder of www.SpiritualParenting.com and
author of *10 Principles for Spiritual Parenting*

"Marvelous! Dr. Reznick is an inspired wizard who has shared with us this book, which is a treasure chest containing nine sparkling gifts of many colors. These tools can be amazingly effective when wielded by our children's powerful imaginations and incredible wisdom."

—Ran D. Anbar, MD, professor of pediatrics and
medicine at SUNY Upstate Medical University

"This book is a must-read for parents and pediatric health-care professionals who want to help their children cope with stressful life events. *The Power of Your Child's Imagination* offers parents an opportunity to partner with their child and guide them in creative problem solving. Dr. Reznick provides the reader with heartwarming scenarios that demonstrate children's ability to use their imagination in creating their own healing."

—Myra Martz Huth, PhD, RN, assistant vice president at the
Center for Professional Excellence at Research and Evidence-Based
Practice at Cincinnati Children's Hospital Medical Center

continued . . .

"Families commonly ask me for ways to help their child cope with stress and anxiety. After reading *The Power of Your Child's Imagination*, I feel that I am better equipped to assuage their concerns. Dr. Reznick lays out nine simple and fun steps that anyone can follow to help their child cope with life's toughest moments. The book not only teaches invaluable lessons but takes the reader on a wonderful journey that is whimsical and fun—how could talking to animal friends, wizards, and even your own toes not be? As I learned how to tap into these magical imaginary worlds I found myself daydreaming, actually alleviating my own day's stress. I think every parent and child can grow by utilizing Dr. Reznick's techniques."

—Scott W. Cohen, MD, FAAP, pediatrician, author of *Eat, Sleep, Poop,*
and cofounder Beverly Hills Pediatrics

"Dr. Reznick's book is an invaluable gift that offers self-care tools that create a ripple effect of healing for parents, children, and the generations to come."

—Terry Reed, RN, MS, HN-BC, codirector of Beyond Ordinary Nursing
and coauthor of *Guided Imagery and Beyond*

"Dr. Reznick has given us all a treasure trove of gems brilliantly designed with heart, care, and wisdom. Each of her nine tools is sure to be used in much the same way as an artist would use the primary colors on her palette to create a masterpiece of success and joy. The rewards are received as soon as you open the book, open your heart, and receive the inherent gifts of unlimited imagination."

—Joyce C. Mills, PhD, LLC, founder of the StoryPlay Center
and coauthor of *Therapeutic Metaphors for Children and the Child Within*

"The tools offered by Dr. Reznick are lovely, effective, and very user-friendly—parents will find the tools and their applications to be very helpful in guiding their children toward mastery in helping themselves."

—Daniel P. Kohen, MD, FAAP, director of the Developmental-Behavioral
Pediatrics Program; professor at the University of Minnesota;
and past president of the American Board of Medical Hypnosis

"Learning to care for oneself, particularly in times of stress, is a key ingredient of emotional intelligence. Dr. Reznick has written a clear and concise blueprint for parents to teach their children how to use their imaginations to cope with both common and uncommon problems. She has created a simple format that nearly every parent can follow and nearly every child will enjoy. I would particularly recommend this book for children with anxiety disorders and fears. The nine tools that form the foundation of the book would be invaluable in teaching children emotional management."

—Lawrence E. Shapiro, PhD, author of
How to Raise a Child with a High EQ

"Dr. Reznick's wonderful book provides an innovative approach to help children work through stressful times. *The Power of Your Child's Imagination* guides parents using practical tools to allow children to discover their potential and explore the inner tools we all possess. An important addition to your parenting library!"

—Lauren Feder, MD, author of *Natural Baby and Childcare* and
The Parents' Concise Guide to Childhood Vaccinations

"The ability to imagine, visualize, and create is becoming increasingly important in our changing world. These are skills children will need to cope and achieve success in the future. This is truly a book that prepares children for the future. I highly recommend it for both educators and parents."

—Robert W. Reasoner, retired school superintendent and
president of the International Council for Self-Esteem

"Finally a guide for parents that moves beyond child psychology and organized religion as guideposts for ensuring a child's emotional health and moral compass. In *The Power of Your Child's Imagination*, Dr. Reznick gives us the tools to access and care for the very essence of our children's being: their soul. A must for any parent who knows that fortifying our children's inner resources is the deepest expression of our love for them." —Vivian Glyck, author of *The Tao of Poop* and founder of
www.JustLikeMyChild.org

continued . . .

"I thoroughly enjoyed *The Power of Your Child's Imagination*, and I believe that parents and health-care professionals alike will find this book an invaluable resource and guide that offers simple tools to help children cope with stress and anxiety by unleashing the power of their own imagination to feel strong and confident. I've used Dr. Reznick's CD, *Discovering Your Special Place*, with many hundreds of my patients over the years, with wonderful benefit to the children and their families. Her new book adds an important dimension...it empowers parents to participate directly in helping their children and, at the same time, it will painlessly remodel and enhance their parenting skills."

—Jim Tipton, MD, pediatric gastroenterology
at Kaiser Permanente, Los Angeles

"This unique and groundbreaking book takes us deeply into the inner worlds of children. Majestic in its simplicity, classic in its wisdom, this book shows how to be the best parent, teaching children the tools through imagery to take charge of their own lives in the greatest way possible. We highly recommend it."

—Charles D. Leviton, EdD, and Patti Leviton, MA,
founders of *Synergy Seminars*

The POWER of YOUR CHILD'S Imagination

How to Transform Stress and Anxiety into Joy and Success

CHARLOTTE REZNICK, PhD

A PERIGEE BOOK

A PERIGEE BOOK
Published by the Penguin Group
Penguin Group (USA) Inc.
375 Hudson Street, New York, New York 10014, USA
Penguin Group (Canada), 90 Eglinton Avenue East, Suite 700, Toronto, Ontario M4P 2Y3, Canada
(a division of Pearson Penguin Canada Inc.)
Penguin Books Ltd., 80 Strand, London WC2R 0RL, England
Penguin Group Ireland, 25 St. Stephen's Green, Dublin 2, Ireland (a division of Penguin Books Ltd.)
Penguin Group (Australia), 250 Camberwell Road, Camberwell, Victoria 3124, Australia
(a division of Pearson Australia Group Pty. Ltd.)
Penguin Books India Pvt. Ltd., 11 Community Centre, Panchsheel Park, New Delhi—110 017, India
Penguin Group (NZ), 67 Apollo Drive, Rosedale, North Shore 0632, New Zealand
(a division of Pearson New Zealand Ltd.)
Penguin Books (South Africa) (Pty.) Ltd., 24 Sturdee Avenue, Rosebank, Johannesburg 2196,
South Africa

Penguin Books Ltd., Registered Offices: 80 Strand, London WC2R 0RL, England

While the author has made every effort to provide accurate telephone numbers and Internet addresses at the time of publication, neither the publisher nor the author assumes any responsibility for errors, or for changes that occur after publication. Further, the publisher does not have any control over and does not assume any responsibility for author or third-party websites or their content.

First edition: August 2009

Library of Congress Cataloging-in-Publication Data

Reznick, Charlotte.
    The power of your child's imagination : how to transform stress and anxiety into joy and success / Charlotte Reznick.
      p. cm.
    "A Perigee book."
    Includes bibliographical references and index.
    ISBN 978-0-399-53507-9
    1. Imagery (Psychology) in children.   2. Stress in children.   3. Stress management in children.
4. Anxiety in children.   5. Interpersonal relations in children.   I. Title.
    BF723.I47.R74 2009
    649'.64—dc22   2009014078

PRINTED IN THE UNITED STATES OF AMERICA

10   9   8   7   6   5   4   3   2

Most Perigee books are available at special quantity discounts for bulk purchases for sales promotions, premiums, fund-raising, or educational use. Special books, or book excerpts, can also be created to fit specific needs. For details, write: Special Markets, Penguin Group (USA) Inc., 375 Hudson Street, New York, New York 10014.

CONTENTS

*For all the children who have touched my heart
and taught me so much.*

ACKNOWLEDGMENTS

There are so many people I wish to thank; without their heartfelt support, this book would have never been written. I am grateful to you all.

Jane and Ronald Deeley, who have always been my rock and my inspiration. They helped me hold on to my dream with their unfathomable love, and believed in me when I didn't believe in myself. Thank you for those 1:00 a.m. phone calls across the globe! Mimi Sells, my beloved friend who, twenty years ago, sat with me and played with chapter titles. Dreams really do come true!

My friends, family, colleagues, and health practitioners for their care, faith, and valued suggestions, from those early days of talking about my desire to write this book, through the years of actual writing. Ron Alexander; Scott Alexander; Patricia Amrhein; Michele Arroyo; Claire Austin; Tom Bolduc; David Bressler; Pat Broeske; Kay Calvin; Jack Canfield; Carol Channel; Phyllis Chase; Lindy and Matt Davidson; Felice Dunas; Linda Eisenberg; Virginia and Mike Fawcett; Gayle Gale; Philip Goldberg; Glenn and Kendra Gorlitsky; Leryn, Brienne, and Garett Gorlitsky; Susan Graysen; Eileen Hearn; Ping Ho; Eric Jacobson; Joyce Jacobson; Harvey Karp; Cathy Kaye; Patricia Lewis; Sid Levin; Valerie Maxwell; Darlene Mininni; Judith Orloff; Emily Putterman; Robert Reasoner; David and Susan Reznick; Stephen and Shelly Reznick; Andy Sells; Lisa Sloan; Karin Solo; Sandy Stern; Marty Rossman; Zee Zee and Karen Sussan; all my meditation group buddies; and of course, my dear friends in my own "Special Place" on the beaches of Menorca, Spain.

Deborah Edler Brown, for her generous heart, unending support, and poetic editing skills. Deb, I couldn't have done this without you! Susan Golant, my very first writing teacher at UCLA, who encouraged me from the start, and who resurfaced to help slash and cut when it was most needed.

Lynn Franklin, my literary agent, whose steady, clear, and calm style guided me through the world of publishing. Maria Gagliano, my editor at Perigee, for her keen eye and kind manner in asking the right questions to make this a better book. John Duff, my publisher at Perigee, whose commitment to this book allows you to read it now.

And finally, my deep appreciation for the pediatricians and parents who entrusted me with the hearts and minds of their patients and children—it has been an honor, and I have learned so much. Thank you.

Introduction

The Power of a Child's Imagination

★ Imagine your frustrated four-year-old calming his anger with a special "Balloon Breath." What if your seven-year-old's own heart could teach her to love herself no matter what? Picture your fourth grader visualizing an ice blue pillow to cool his hot headaches. Or your worried eleven-year-old improving her concentration by consulting a personal wizard to assist with homework.

Imagine if every child could tap into an inexhaustible source of strength and wisdom when life gets tough. Think of how their lives would transform.

Growing up today is harder than ever as kids cope with unprecedented stress. The nightly news is a parade of bleak images—natural disasters, terrorism, street violence, and war—making our children feel unsafe. People are more isolated; extended families aren't the haven they once were. Troubles that challenge adults—divorce, addiction, and financial worries—translate into conflict at home as kids absorb their parents' woes. Add to that the traditional hurts and challenges of childhood—academic and social pressure, schoolyard bullies, the death of a pet or dear grandparent—and it's not surprising that more kids are acting out or simply shutting down.

Child psychiatrists and researchers in the United States and abroad report an escalation of regressive behaviors, a rise in fear of everyday activities such as going to sleep or school, and an increase in anxiety masquerading as physical ailments such as headaches, stomachaches, tics, and fatigue—all in the last decade.[1]

Children's positive views of themselves are also at risk. According to one study, while 60 percent of third and fourth graders reported that they liked themselves, by eleventh grade, only 46 percent of boys and 29 percent of girls felt that way.[2] Other studies now warn that the very quality we want our kids to have—good self-esteem—might twist them into narcissistic, "only thinking about me" adults.[3] The conflicting research confuses parents and professionals alike. We do know that low self-esteem in children can lead to poor life choices such as truancy, drug use, teen pregnancy, or even thoughts of suicide.[4]

And while computers and technology have no doubt enhanced communication and research, they have also disturbed our natural sense of time. Everyone expects instant results: Fast food. Email. Text messages. We've simply lost patience, allowing no time to stop and think, rest and relax, or slow down and feel. No time remains to develop the emotional skills necessary for a balanced, successful, and happy life.

All this can make raising healthy, well-adjusted kids feel like an overwhelming—if not impossible—task. How can you guide and protect your children when the odds seem so daunting? When you're working so hard and your stress is sky high? When there's rarely time to work out problems as they arise? When life changes so quickly? When no one taught you how? The answer is to stop looking *out* for answers and start looking *in*. Into the heart of your child. Into his or her mind and imagination.

Imagination Is Not Just Child's Play

Adults have long used imagery and visualization to improve creativity, physical and mental health, as well as sports and professional performance. Whether it's an athlete's focused reverie before stepping on the field, or a cancer patient's mental image of immune cells gobbling up a tumor, studies have shown that guided imagery relieves stress, reduces illness, lessens pain, improves performance, and alleviates anxiety and sleep disorders.[5]

It is equally effective with children. Researchers around the world have demonstrated the positive effects of relaxation training and imagery on children and teens. Academic achievement and sports performance improve. Behavioral difficulties decrease, as do the number and the intensity of illnesses and symptoms. Even the required levels of medication for asthma and postoperative pain relief can come down.[6]

As a child educational psychologist and associate clinical professor of psychology at UCLA, I have long believed in the healing power of a child's imagination. In fact, I built my career on it. For more than twenty-five years, my life has focused on the rich internal world of children, a magical place where wise and creative answers reside. I began this work after being assigned to an inner-city school in South Central Los Angeles while still a fresh, naïve psychologist. On a balmy September day, I drove into the poorest area of the city, armed only with my ideals, a degree from USC, and a deep desire to help kids. The streets were filled with graffiti. So many stores were boarded up, burned, or had broken windows, the neighborhood resembled a war zone.

In the very first classroom, I was introduced as the *nice new counselor* who would help the students with their problems. I could feel their piercing eyes ask, "Who are you, lady? What are you doing here, anyway?" I thought I heard a muffled laugh. Tough, bulky Jerome, with a two-inch scar over his right eye, scoffed and went on punching his neighbor. Later I learned his dad had "accidentally" cut him in a drunken rage. Mercedes, sporting a brightly flowered but soiled dress, stared at me blankly.

Who was I to attempt to reach out to these children, whose life experiences were so different from mine? How could I help them reach inside and find a space that was filled with light and laughter? Was it possible for them to find some inner peace? Could they learn to believe in themselves enough to create a future?

The conventional counseling practices I'd been taught didn't work here. These kids were angry, depressed, abused, lonely, detached, doing poorly in school, and generally feeling miserable. How could they learn in school when they were worried about how they were going to eat, or who was going to "beat up" on them? How could they focus on academics if they were fretting about their parents' fighting, drug use, or whereabouts at night? Desperation led me to explore avenues beyond traditional behavioral therapy. I had to use my imagination. And theirs.

I first discovered the power of imagination attending a state psychological conference in those early years. Workshop leaders had asked us to draw a picture of a favorite place. Mine looked like a six-year-old had drawn it. Then they asked us to close our eyes and led us through the most delightful inner journey to a lush, peaceful meadow, filled with tall, scented pines, shimmering emerald plants, and beautiful blooming flowers. A gentle stream trickled nearby. Listening to the rich evocative language, I was transported. They invited us to draw again. What a difference! This time my drawing was lovely, and it actually captured what I imagined. That tangible change—from a childlike scrawl to an expressive picture in a matter of minutes—caught my attention.

The instructors then recounted the success they'd had with imagery techniques in a school district aptly named "Paradise Unified." Academic achievement on standardized tests increased; behavioral referrals diminished. Teachers reported students were better at calming themselves and staying on task.[7] The hairs on my skin stood up. Could visualization actually help the distressed kids I worked with? On an intellectual and visceral level, this made sense.

I began to read every book, take every course, attend every lecture, and meet every person I could find who had anything to do with imagery and visualization. Devouring it all, I made it my own, learning what worked and what didn't with *my* kids; what would touch their hearts, what would shut them down.

Imagery did something that conventional therapies could not. Bypassing the natural defenses of the logical brain, it allowed children to go directly to the intuitive part of themselves and let their heart speak. Instead of *talking about* feelings, they were invited to *experience* their feelings and express them in pictures. Their images told a deeper truth than these children could say in words, and gave them a discovery process that felt more like a game than a chore. The answers they found to their problems were more effective than any advice or instruction coming from the adults around them, including me.

I took the basic tenets of imagery work—that you can engage with pictures conjured by your mind and intuition to bring awareness to emotions and find solutions to issues *ordinary thinking* doesn't supply—wove them with traditional breathing, meditation, and the focused awareness and suggestions of self-hypnosis techniques, included sound psychological principles, and created a novel approach that applied to all aspects of a child's daily life.

And by exploring and trusting in the power of my own creative imagination, backed by the research and experiences of colleagues, I learned how to help these children help themselves. Child by child, imagination to imagination, heart to heart—I was able to reach them.

South Central was the testing ground. If these children could summon hope from despair and learn to help themselves, then these imagery Tools could work for everyone. And they did. One student tracked me down years later to tell me she was now student body president of her high school. "Every time I'm about to get up in front of the assembly, I remember an image I learned with you in fifth grade," she told me. "I see myself standing on top of the mountain of success."

Those early explorations developed into a full program that includes nine specific Tools I have taught in public and private schools, to clients from all walks of life, and in professional trainings and workshops around the world. They are:

1 The Balloon Breath—The Way In
2 Discovering Your Special Place
3 Meeting a Wise Animal Friend
4 Encountering a Personal Wizard
5 Receiving Gifts from Inner Guides
6 Checking In with Heart and Belly
7 Talking to Toes and Other Body Parts
8 Using Color for Healing
9 Tapping into Energy

These Tools facilitate a child's inward journey to that deep place sometimes called the subconscious or unconscious. They are easy-to-use, whimsical, and remarkably effective. Each touches a world of metaphor, creating a waking dream. These images help children direct their attention to problems and symptoms they want to change or to potentials they want to develop.

Used together, the Tools teach children a way to harness inner wisdom to understand, heal, and ultimately love themselves. While parents and children often come to me with specific concerns—anxiety, anger, stress-related physical complaints, or simply because they want to build strong inner resources—I see these issues as the key to opening that first door. Once a child learns to use imagination techniques, she can transfer these skills to many other life challenges.

Equally important, these are Tools children can learn to use on their own. How often do we (parents and therapists alike) look to others for a quick fix? Rarely do we trust our own wisdom, let alone the wisdom of our children. Yet, with just a little guidance, our kids can gain access to the answers for most of life's questions within themselves. They learn best when they solve their own problems. As the saying goes, "Give a man a fish, and he eats for a day. Teach a man to fish, and he eats for a lifetime."

I wrote *The Power of Your Child's Imagination* to teach *you* to teach your child how to fish . . . for the food of the soul, of the growing Self, with the tools of imagination. My hope is to create a world in which every child has the tools to heal herself and realize her dreams. And that still happens child by child, heart by heart, and now, parent by parent.

This book is a toolbox for possibility and change. You'll help your kids use imagination to access their natural strengths and wisdom, and deal with their problems. The techniques are so simple—yet so powerful—that even a child as young as four can use them. More than power tools, they are tools that *em*power.

How to Read This Book

The Power of Your Child's Imagination is divided into two sections. Part One, "The Tools," sets the groundwork for building your child's inner resources. In Chapter 1, you will find ways to help "hook" your kids' enthusiasm, questions that draw them in, and techniques to calm any hesitation for this new experience.

In Chapter 2, I elaborate on each of the Nine Tools in detail. This is the heart of the program. Simple instructions and sample scripts will guide you in teaching each Tool to your child. I call these *foundation Tools* because they are not only the foundation of this program and book, but also the foundation for a lifetime of self-sufficiency and self-growth.

Music, drawing, and writing can enhance the problem solving that imagery inspires, acting like a booster pack for the Nine Tools. In Chapter 3, you'll explore how to use and combine these skills.

Chapter 4 is for you—the big kids. Although we all want to do our best, sometimes it just doesn't happen. This chapter shows how the Nine Tools can enhance your interactions with your children. They can be adapted so that you can experience less personal stress and more freedom to be creative in your parenting. My top ten list, "What Kids Most Want and Need from Their Parents," will ensure your success as a role model in teaching these skills to your children. Put into practice, the Top Ten will also result in happier, healthier kids and a thriving family. There is also a special guided relaxation script to nurture your own spirit.

Part Two, "Putting the Tools to Work," is a user-friendly guide that shows you how to apply the Nine Tools to eight common life challenges:

- How your child can be his own best friend
- Reducing stress-induced ailments
- Overcoming fears and feeling safe
- Dealing with bedtime issues
- Coping with loss
- Handling hurt, anger, and frustration
- Achieving success at school and play
- Living peacefully with family and friends

Each chapter in this section demonstrates, step-by-step, how to apply the Tools to these common childhood issues, sharing stories of children who have used imagination to turn their lives around.* I also include Quick Tips, Sample Scripts, Easy Hints, and lots of How-To For You ideas to help you apply these skills to your own family and situation. There are even Backtrack Alerts, which anticipate those moments when something seems to be going wrong. I'll explain how these are just part of this new learning process.

Every chapter ends with a specific guided imagery you can read to your child before or after your imagination sessions, or you can order a recorded CD version in my voice from my website, www .ImageryForKids.com. These mini-journeys deepen the healing experience. The scripts help your child relax, feel safe, and gain confidence around the problem as he progresses in this visual process toward self-discovery.

The appendix is designed for the professionals who shape a child's world: teachers, doctors, nurses, counselors, therapists, and all those who have daily opportunities to offer a positive influence on children. It suggests how the principles of this program can be incorporated into your working world.

I designed *The Power of Your Child's Imagination* to be both a reading book and a how-to manual. You can read it straight through or go directly to a relevant chapter. If you do choose to turn to a specific problem chapter, then I recommend that you read Chapters 1 and 2 first, as they introduce and explain all Nine Tools and how to apply them.

As you follow this program, you will be well equipped to offer your children the skills that build self-esteem, emotional self-sufficiency, and resilience. You will feel more confident as you

---

*Note: The names and identifying characteristics of the children and families mentioned in this book and the details of their stories have been changed or combined to protect their privacy.

teach your kids to solve many of their own problems. And as you encourage them to find their own answers, you will find that you actually create more trust, intimacy, and joy in your relationship with them.

These Nine Tools are adaptable to all ages, and their benefits accumulate over time. These are not just tools for childhood; they are tools for life. In the words of one wise eight-year-old, "Your imagination can help you heal."

PART ONE

THE TOOLS

CHAPTER 1

The Way Out Is Through the Inside

Harnessing Your Child's Imagination

> **Imagery helps me relax and makes me feel smart. I love to imagine.**
>
> —Libby, age nine

★ Six-year-old Alec couldn't go to bed alone. Every night, his mom sat with him until the anxious boy fell asleep. Then she would tiptoe out, hoping not to wake him. If she left sooner, he would tremble and beg her to stay. When she asked about his fears, his response was surprisingly precocious. "I believe in ghosts and goblins," he said. "I think they come through walls. I think they're real. I'm a little kid, and I have a big imagination."

Mind and imagination are powerful forces, especially in a growing child. They are catalysts for so much more than bedtime fears. The stories a child tells herself, what she thinks and imagines, determine how she reacts to the events in her life and, essentially, who she becomes. Consider any problem your child is facing right now—struggles at school or with friends, sorrow over a loss, jealousy over a new baby, physical illness—and you'll find much of her suffering stems from how she thinks about it.

For a child to thrive in the world, he must thrive inside. We spend so much time on the externals—how children behave, how they handle their bodies and interact with others—that we rarely address the inside places where personality and imagination, mind and heart, reside. The places where a Self is born. Yet the same skills adults use to improve creative and professional performance can help your child discover increased health, confidence, and self-esteem.

Like Alec, your child has a big imagination. We're going to make it an ally, tapping his inner knowledge to help him heal himself and realize his dreams. Simply discovering that he *has* his own wisdom will be empowering. Developing the habit of listening to it and trusting it will profoundly shape how he meets life's challenges.

"But he's just a boy," you might be thinking. "How much can really be accomplished through a child's own knowing?" A lot. Each of us has a wiser self, an internal compass that seems to "know" more than we do. We don't always listen to that little voice inside our head, but it's there. I've heard it speak to children as young as four years old, giving them sound advice and new perspective on their troubles.

And a shift in that internal world can change the outer one, as star athletes confirm. They have long used imagination to prepare for the "mental game" as seriously as the physical one. If these techniques can affect the outcome of a sporting event, think what they can do in life's major marathon—growing up.

The fact that you are reading this book—either to address a specific issue or to increase your parenting skills—tells me that imagery has captured your imagination. The question now is how to get your child to play along.

Engaging Your Child

How you introduce imagery and the Nine Tools to your child depends on her age and personality, her concerns, and her experience with problem solving. However you broach the subject, do so lightly. Imagery is fun—that's what makes it effective. Even if your child is working through specific issues, you don't need to make it only about "her problem." Anxious kids often worry about their anxiety; too much attention might worsen it. So skip the front door approach and slip in sideways. You're holding the key to an astonishing place—your child's inner world. Enter gently.

Invite Imagination to Dinner

Children use their imaginations every day—alone and with friends—as they play games and make up stories. But it's seen as "kid stuff," set apart from the practical and problematic worlds of school and family life. A gentle way to introduce imagery is simply to invite your child's imagination into your day-to-day conversations. Play "What If." For instance, several paintings hang in my office: a flower-filled meadow, a wooded path, and celestial clouds. When I start treating a child, I often ask, "If you were to go into one of those paintings, which would you choose?" This warm-up invites his imagination into my office, a place it has never been. You can do the same at meals, bedtime, or in the car. Use anything around you: a picture, a book, a billboard. What would it be like to be inside it? Start with objects you can see, especially with little kids. Then, with eyes open, have your child imagine things he can't see: a lizard crawling up the wall or a flower growing in an empty pot. What does it look like? Starting with open eyes gives him a feeling of control, a safer way to try a new experience.

When he's ready, invite him to close his eyes and suggest items that stimulate the senses. Can he recall the rhythm of his favorite song? The look and taste of a great dessert? Maybe he's petting a puppy or kitten, or dipping his feet in a mountain stream. What does *that* feel like? You can also try the "biting into a lemon" trick—just thinking about it makes our lips pucker. Our brain interprets all these images as real.

Now move into pure imagination: What would it be like to explore Africa? What would your teddy bear say if he could talk?

Once your child is used to sharing his imagination with *you*, it will be easier to use it with problems and dreams.

Make It About What Matters

Address your child's unique needs and desires. What does she complain about? Long for? How would she like her life to improve or change? This is a natural next step from the imagination games above. She doesn't even have to acknowledge problems. Watching and listening will tell you plenty. If she has an issue that is clearly on the table—a fight with a friend, a poor grade, or an upsetting baseball game—you can weave her concerns into your conversations and ask questions you know will elicit a positive response:

- Do you want more friends?
- Would you like to make learning easier?
- Do you want to improve in sports?
- Would you like to get along better with your sister?

These questions tap into inner wishes that imagery has the power to grant. They open the door for you to say, "Your imagination is a great place to start."

However, some kids benefit from addressing concerns directly. You might say, "I know this problem has been bothering you for a while. Can you imagine it improving?" If your child says no, because he thinks it's impossible, applaud his honesty. Then ask, "If it *were* possible, if it *could* get better, would you be interested?" Stop there. If this whets his curiosity, great. Give him a few days, then let him know you've been thinking about him and his issue. Would he consider learning new ways to address it? If so, you're in. Praise his adventurousness. Tell him you believe in him, that you'll help him find answers, and that he'll learn how to accomplish his goals.

Make It a Game

With younger ones, ages four to six, a playful approach may work better: "Mommy has a fun game for us. It's called the Balloon Breath. Let me show you how it goes." You don't need to address problems at this point. Deep breathing will naturally calm him, no matter what his troubles, and get him ready to find creative solutions to many "games" of life—from academics to sports. From there, you can move into more imagination games, right down the Nine Tools list.

Address a Crisis

Sometimes you can't wait another minute. If your child is in enough emotional or physical distress, she'll be motivated to try anything. That's when I suggest the Fast Track approach. First, stay positive. Reassure her that this problem won't last forever. You might not know how it will change or when, but together you will find solutions. Then take her into the peaceful breathing of the Balloon Breath (Tool 1). It's easy to learn and will immediately relieve some anxiety. When she's calmer, show her how to find a Special Place, an imaginary refuge discovered through Tool 2. Whether or not the large issue can be quickly resolved, knowing that she can quiet herself and find an inner sanctuary will likely ease her suffering. By then, you'll be well into the process.

Respect Resistance

Occasionally children resist the idea of imagery work. Their imagination might be an old friend from play, but the idea of using it to solve problems is new, and the unfamiliar can be suspect. Point out those times when your child used his imagination to overcome challenges and didn't realize it. Like when he imagined riding around the block with his buddies even before he learned to ride a bike. Or she imagined meeting and playing with new friends well before the school year began. Such examples can motivate them to try this novel approach.

If your child still declines, don't press; you'll only inspire rebellion. Validate his feelings and mirror what he tells you by using his words or rephrasing them. A simple, nonjudgmental observation such as, "I hear that you don't care if you get bad grades. I wonder if that's tough on you?" can move a child's heart. If he feels you understand his experience, that you are on *his* team, he's more likely to consider other possibilities.

Kids sometimes hesitate facing their problems because they're afraid they can't be overcome. This fear of failure keeps kids—and grown-ups—safe in old habits. Embarrassment can also make them waver. Children may alternate between interest and dismissal ("That sounds dumb!"), or they may ask questions but avoid actually learning the Tools. These are natural reactions that you should respect. Your child needs to trust that you honor his feelings, whatever they are. In fact, the more room he has to say no, the more likely he is to say yes. Let him know you are always there if he changes his mind.

And certain older children may be interested in trying the Tools, but not with you. In this case, consider recording the sample scripts so your child can listen to them alone. Or order online *The Power of Your Child's Imagination* CD—a recording of the scripts in this book. Encourage her to draw or write about her experiences; this might start a conversation between you. If it doesn't, a well-timed and placed Post-It note supporting her and praising her efforts can mean a lot. Either way, she'll benefit from the work.

Teaching the Tools

When I work with a child, I have a luxury afforded few parents: a fixed schedule and an uninterrupted hour. But imagination work is flexible and can be slipped into odd moments throughout the day. Bedtime is often when kids let down their guard and share how they feel. The car is another great spot; it's amazing how many openings come when a child is lulled by the rhythm of the road. Once you're engaged, you'll find many quick practice moments in the natural structure of your days.

Teaching the Tools, however, requires some time and focus. This is new material for both of you, and you'll want ample space to get comfortable with it.

So how do you start? First, take a deep breath and release your expectations. Caring parents—the kind who buy books like this—want to get it "right." But there's no such animal. Not here. You're entering the realm of the imagination where anything is possible and everything is okay. The instructions and scripts are guidelines, not formulas. As you work with the Tools, you'll eventually make them your own. Trust your intuition and creativity. That's no more than you're asking of your child.

Read the Nine Tools in Chapter 2 a few times to familiarize yourself with them. Practice with a partner or friend. You don't have to memorize the scripts, just read from the book. Plan on teaching one Tool at a time—even part of one—adding the next as need or intuition dictate.

Set Aside Imagine Time

Expect to spend fifteen to thirty minutes per Tool, depending on your child's temperament and which Tool you're introducing.

Younger children have shorter attention spans, so you might need to break the "lesson" into two short segments. Or, you might want more time in case they get distracted and need to be pulled back in. There is no wrong way to do this. But do try to give yourself enough time to teach the skill, practice it, and talk, draw, or write afterward. After one or two sessions, you'll know how much time you need for your individual child.

Create a Soothing Environment

Play soft background music to create a calm atmosphere. Pick a place where you won't be interrupted. Some kids like to sit in a chair or lie on the floor, while others prefer their bed. Location doesn't matter, so long as your child feels comfy. In fact, the more relaxed her body is, the deeper into imagination she'll go.

Introduce Today's Tool

Spend a minute letting your child know what to expect from each new Tool. It's as simple as saying, "Today we're going to go to a Special Place." Then explain what that is. With little kids, you might also draw pictures. Answer any questions before you begin.

Settle In

Once your child is comfortable, encourage her to close her eyes; it will block distractions and help her connect inside. If this makes her uneasy, don't push; but if she can shut her eyes, even for several seconds, she'll experience a deeper response. You might suggest that if outside thoughts intrude—about school, friends, or sports—she can put them in an imaginary balloon, to float away or pick up later, and return her focus to her breathing. And always remind her to signal you if anything makes her uncomfortable.

Begin the Journey

Scripts and exercises for all the foundation Tools are provided in Chapter 2. You can read them as written—slowly and softly, with ample pauses—or paraphrase them, adjusting the vocabulary or length to match your child's age and understanding. With young children, a few sentences might do. You can add more next time. As you lead your child through each script, let him know he can change anything he dislikes. One girl started traveling down a dark tunnel too fast. When she told me, I suggested she slow herself down and use a flashlight to help her see where she was going.

Whichever Tool you're teaching, start with the Balloon Breath. It creates relaxed concentration that facilitates the others.

Weigh the Value of Interaction

When you first introduce each Tool, guide your child through the short journey without conversation, letting him go as deep as possible without having to respond. Just have him lift a hand or finger if he wants to say something; that puts him in control of the interaction. You can talk about his experience when the meditation is over.

As you both get comfortable, after a few times with the script, allow yourself to alter it based on a simple running conversation about his changing experience, with his eyes still closed. He might say he's cold in his Special Place; ask him if there's something there that could warm him—if not, offer an imaginary blanket or heater. He might get a message but not be able to read it; find out if someone could translate; if need be, suggest a light to reveal the letters. His reactions will suggest how to adjust the journey.

And some children want more interaction with you from the start. In these cases, lead your child through, step-by-step right away. Experiment with both methods.

Share the Discovery

After her imagination journey, invite your child to share what happened. Let her know she can reveal feelings and discoveries without repercussion. Find out what she still needs. If something seems unresolved—a gift left in a corner, a feeling unheard or unanswered—have her close her eyes and go back to resolve it. Some kids, however, just aren't talkers. Writing and drawing (Chapter 3) are great outlets for them. And if they want to keep their experience private, well, that's fine, too.

Practicing the Tools

As your child learns all Nine Tools, you can subtly introduce them into daily life. The beauty of imagination work is that it uses as much time as you have. Transitions make natural breaks: after school, mealtime, before homework, in the car, before bed. These are perfect moments to take a few minutes, quickly center, and check inside. Upsets are also opportunities. Perhaps world events have distressed your child. Talk about peace beginning within, and practice the Balloon Breath to remember what *Peaceful* feels like.

Kids frequently adopt the language you use, whether it's the names of the Tools or the way you make suggestions. Use positive, affirming words. Tell your child what you want him to do, not what you don't want. Instead of "Don't be nervous," try "Be brave."

Instead of "Stop blinking," say, "Let's relax." And don't be surprised when your child asks for *his* Tools by name.

Clear Goals and Real Results

The goal of the Nine Tools is always to find a positive solution to the problem at hand. If your child isn't sleeping well, the goal is to sleep serenely. If she's doing poorly in school, the goal is to improve her grades. And if he's wetting the bed, the goal is dry sleep. Sometimes you might have multiple goals, baby steps toward the ideal result. A child who doesn't know how to express feelings might work toward first being aware of what she is feeling, then expressing her feelings with you, with the end goal of expressing them with her friends. Clear goals are most useful when a problem is obvious to your child and you both agree on a desired result: a pain-free tummy, courage at the doctor's office, overcoming stage fright.

However, clear goals may not always be the best starting point. Not when children see the problem differently than you do. Andrew's parents viewed him as angry and fighting a lot at home. But this nine-year-old didn't think he was fighting. "Stop fighting" was his parents' goal, not his. I didn't even address it initially. Instead, I asked Andrew what would make his life easier. He felt his brother picked on him and wanted it to stop. Since that was *his* goal, that's what we talked about—and used his imagination for. Andrew was then willing to consider how his own behavior toward his brother interfered with reaching his goal.

The Nine Tools can help your child achieve the goals you have for her, but only when they are also *her* goals. By first understanding and respecting her goals, then finding some common ground, you can steer her in a direction you both value.

Launch Pad for Conversation

One of the wonderful things about using the Nine Tools in a family setting is the way they can open up new channels of communication. Although much of the work takes place inside your child's imagination, as you guide him through a private journey, it doesn't begin or end there. There are many opportunities for conversation, discovery, and connection along the way.

Talking Up the Tools: The process of introducing imagery and the Tools to your child is more than a sales pitch. It's an opportunity to relate in a new way, one in which her playful inner world is a valued part of her daily life. By taking her flights of fancy seriously and inviting them into conversation, you plant seeds of confidence and self-respect. Unless you have a child in distress, take your time with this. Enjoy an unstructured exploration of her imagination. Play along. When was the last time you gave your imagination the respect it deserves?

Exploring Issues: To make full use of the Tools, it's important to really talk and listen to your child. His worries and complaints are keys to his growth. So are your casual chats with him, the little things he says and does. I always talk with kids before they begin the inner work. I ask about their day, their life, their desires, and I base our inner exploration on what they tell me and, sometimes, on what they don't. One ten-year-old came to me right before New Year's. I asked about her accomplishments in the last year and what changes she'd like to make in the next. She wanted more friends and better grades in school. But although she was constantly biting her nails to the quick, that never made the list. It hadn't occurred to her. When

I asked if she'd like to learn to let her nails grow, she said yes, and we began to address it. Had she said no, we would have still entered a meaningful dialogue. Perhaps we would have discussed why not and what biting her nails meant to her. By listening to your child, with respect for his perceptions and his feelings, you open the door to heart-to-heart conversations that will only strengthen the bond between you.

Negotiating Practical Solutions: As you guide your child through the Nine Tools, you'll learn a lot about the stressors that cause his problems. And while you can't actually make a friend play nicely or return a new baby, you still have lots of power. Listen for the ones you can address, like his too busy schedule or anxiety when you're late, and see how, together, you can create some adjustments to make a difference.

Unraveling the Story: Another important exchange takes place after her inner journeys. By receiving her stories with delight and understanding, you make it safe for her to share feelings and experiences. This lays the groundwork for more openness on her part and a closer connection between you. Although the Tools will teach your child to solve many of her own problems, there will always be situations she'll need your help to resolve. Building trust now paves the way for future cooperation.

Bolstering Her Spirits: Kids expect instant results and can easily get discouraged. If yours becomes impatient and wants to give up, she may fear she's doing this wrong or be frustrated that her life isn't changing faster. Reassure her that any response is fine and that healing takes time. Then take this as an opportunity to talk about persistence. Remind her of a time she had to work hard but finally "got it"—and how great that felt. Tell her stories from your own life. This kind of sharing may inspire her to try again. If not, take a break.

Let her know that you'll check in next week to see how she feels and have a fresh start. The conversation itself might be the healing she needed today.

It's All Improv

Improvisation, whether it's on the stage or in the kitchen, is spontaneous and immediate, and it makes use of whatever is at hand. Imagery is always about improv. No one knows what will surface from your child's imagination—not even he. The same Tools work in radically different situations. And the most surprising discoveries come out of the moment you're in.

Although it will take some time and practice until you and your child are comfortable enough with the Tools and scripts to improvise freely, remember that your child's imagination is just one part of this journey. Your intuition and creativity are the other. Keep your eyes, ears, and heart open for where you can personalize the process.

Tailor the Scripts: Weave in specific suggestions about whatever is bothering your child. For instance, if she's worried her friends won't play with her, adjust the script so that she receives help on how to create a friendlier atmosphere or advice on reaching out. If new concerns arise afterward, as you discuss the imagery, she can always return "inside" for more answers.

Create Your Own Scripts: Once you are comfortable with the rhythm and format of each script, you can add to them, or make up your own imageries to meet the moment.

Change the Order of Tools: I generally introduce the Tools in a specific order, and usually start off with the Balloon Breath. But the real question in my mind is always what is needed *right now*. For a very frightened child, or one with stress-related aches and pains, it might mean Talking to Toes and Other Body Parts (Tool 7), which helps him discover where fear or tension resides. Energy for Healing (Tool 9) may be just the calming place to start with a very agitated child. Then, once he settles down a bit, I can teach him the Balloon Breath. As you get used to using the Nine Tools, they will feel less like steps and more like, well, *tools*. Just like a hammer or wrench, you'll look for the one that matches the problem before you.

Making the Tools Their Own

Most children learn to request and use the Tools on their own, but it doesn't happen at once. Learning new skills takes time. In fact, it takes three to four weeks for the brain to develop a pattern for any new habit. So if your child practices the Balloon Breath with you daily, she may be able to use it by herself in about a month. That's not to say you must do this every day. Only that the more a child practices a skill, the faster she makes it hers.

Learning also occurs in stages. Children first acquire the language of the Tools, the names and the phrases you use to discuss them. So a young child's Animal Friend may advise him to "do the Balloon Breath" well before he understands its full significance. He may simply understand that it's something you value, or be mimicking your advice and encouragement. That's fine. This budding advice from inside empowers him to begin to embrace the Tools as his own.

As they go along, children discover favorite Tools. These are the ones they ask for and learn most easily. How quickly your child uses a Tool without your guidance will also be determined by his age, personality, and what he's taken a special liking to. And, of course, children learn to *use* the Tools long before they *remember* to use them. Remembering is its own skill and requires practice. Think of how many good habits you're trying to acquire, and you'll understand what I mean.

This is not a race or an aptitude test. Your child will learn the Tools with you; he will incorporate them into his life as they become meaningful to him. The real goal is to help him heal and grow. And that can begin immediately.

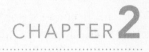

CHAPTER 2

How to Get from Here to There

The breath is the way in.

—*Mateo, age five*

The Nine Core Tools

★ The Nine Core Tools, the foundation of this book, teach a child to use his inner world to navigate the challenges of growing up. If there were "magic beans" you could give your child, these Tools would be them—created by one of the most powerful entities on earth: a young imagination.

The Tools are listed in a particular order, each building upon the next. By teaching them this way, you slowly stretch your child's "imagine muscles" from the familiar—animals, wizards, and gifts— to more abstract notions of feelings, color, and energy. Once you start practicing the Tools, there will be overlap. In Part Two, you'll learn to combine them in a variety of ways to help your child face typical childhood troubles. Relax into this process. It's a lovely journey and works best with a good dose of *play*.

Tool 1. The Balloon Breath—The Way In

If the Nine Tools are the foundation of this program, the Balloon Breath is the *foundation* Tool. It is a deep, diaphragmatic breathing technique that you and your child will return to again and again as you reap its benefits.

Few people actually breathe deeply. Ask someone to, and he'll suck in his belly and puff out his chest, a lot like Superman. But a diaphragmatic breath fills the body like a balloon, from the bottom. It's the belly, not the chest, that rises and falls first. Watch a sleeping baby or puppy and you'll see.

Ancient wisdom and modern research point to the calming effects and health benefits of slow, deep breathing. It's a basic component of meditation, practiced for over 5,000 years across cultures, religions, and within the secular world, and helps people slow down and turn their attention inward. It is also used in hypnosis, facilitating a waking state of focused concentration and increased receptivity to positive directed suggestions.[1]

Once your child masters the Balloon Breath, he will have learned "the way in" to his private world. He'll be in the perfect place to hear his inner voice and make the most of the next eight Tools.

Preparing Yourself

Before you teach the Balloon Breath, explore it for yourself. While this technique can be practiced in any position, at any time or location, it's most easily demonstrated lying down. Get comfortable on a flat surface and place your hands around your navel. Focus your attention two to three inches below it, and breathe slowly and deeply into your lower belly so that it presses into your hands like an inflating balloon. Stay there for a minute or two, feeling its gentle rise and fall. Notice how you feel. Try it sitting and standing. Now you're ready to teach your child.

Preparing Your Child

The simplest way to start is to demonstrate how easy it is. Have your child put her hands on your belly to feel your breath coming in and going out. Then have her try it on her own tummy. With a younger child, you can illustrate with an actual balloon—watch it fill with air and then let it release and soften. Encourage her to think about or imagine the breath going into her nose and down to her belly. This will focus her mind and calm her body.

The Balloon Breath doesn't take long to learn. The sample script will walk your child through it. If she prefers to sit up, make sure she's in a relaxed position with her legs hanging down. It's also okay for her to sit cross-legged on the floor—yoga-style. Repeat the script until she is comfortable with the process, perhaps three times with her eyes open and three more with them closed. After each round, ask how she felt. Was there a difference from one session to the next?

Practice one to three times daily, starting with three breaths and working up to seven to ten (about a minute). After a week, increase her time by one minute every two or three weeks, until you reach five minutes. Remind her when to practice by putting up colorful stickers in places of stress or habit, like the homework desk or by her toothbrush. Whenever she sees one, she can take three more Balloon Breaths. You can, too!

The Balloon Breath

"Imagine blowing up a balloon. Then picture letting the air out slowly, until the balloon goes flat. Can you see it? In a minute, we're going to pretend your stomach is a balloon. You're going to take a deep breath in, all the way down to your lower belly, hold it for a few seconds, then let it go gently.

"Get ready by putting your hands on your belly, about two inches below your belly button. Good.

"Now, take a few minutes to think about your breathing. Take a slow deep breath. Feel it going in and out . . . in and out. That's right. Breathe slowly so your belly and your hands rise and fall. Good.

"Let's breathe in even slower—to the count of one . . . two . . . three.

"Now breathe out just as slowly . . . one . . . two . . . three.

"Take a few minutes to practice . . .

"When you're ready, pay attention to your hands and your feet. Where are they? What are they touching?

"Now open your eyes slowly."

Practice Notes and Variations

A Rainbow Breath: By four, most kids recognize a rainbow and can imagine one quickly. Bring your child close to you and put your hands on his lower belly and back; this will hold him still and give him a place to focus. Suggest he close his eyes and imagine breathing a beautiful rainbow of love into his belly, then imagine filling up his whole body with it.

A Breath Game: The benefits of the Balloon Breath come from breathing deeply and *slowly*. Play a game with your child to see how few breaths she can take in a minute. Time her, and whatever number she reaches, praise her. The new goal is to take fewer breaths next time.

Hold a Beloved Object: Relaxation and concentration can be hard for younger kids, whose bodies simply want to *move*. Even older ones may find stillness to be a challenge. If this is the case, try giving your child a favorite small object to hold. It will give her body something to do while her mind tracks her breathing.

Hand and Body Positions: Once your child is comfortable with the Balloon Breath, consider experimenting with different hand and body positions.[2] Hands are expressive. Just as a clenched fist mimics stress or anger, open palms are receptive and "open-handed." Having a clear purpose for her hands also prevents fidgeting.

- *Cupped hands*: In the sitting position, have your child put her hands in her lap, palms up, with the right hand resting on top of and completely over the left, and thumb tips touching.
- *Open palms*: This restful position can be attained lying down, with the palms facing up at the sides, or sitting, with the back of hands on the knees or on the chair seat.
- *Supported breath*: Touch and relaxation add up to extra comfort in stressful times. Sit behind your child and place your hands on the center of his back at heart level. This will support him as he calms himself with breathing.
- *Twin balloons*: Breathing together is a sweet, intimate activity. Sit cross-legged, facing each other. Rest your palms against each other, with yours face up below his. Do several Balloon Breaths together.

Back to the Body: If the Balloon Breath is the doorway to deep relaxation and reverie, your child's own body is the way back to everyday reality. The script ends with attention to his hands and feet to transition him from a waking dream state back to the concrete world. Feel free to suggest more details, based on the real physical circumstances. For instance, if he's sitting up, "What does the floor feel like under your feet?" Or if he's in bed, "Notice how the blanket feels under your hands." It grounds him in his body and brings him gently back into the present moment.

How Kids Use It

Anxiety permeated Enzo's life. This nine-year-old was scared to go to school because he worried terrible things would happen to his mom while he was gone. He was afraid to sleep when his dad took business trips because he kept dreaming of plane crashes. In short, he resisted spending any time away from his parents. Of all the Tools that Enzo learned, the Balloon Breath most calmed his anxious thoughts. Then he could reason with himself and begin to logically release his fears. Within three months, he went from a fearful child, glued to his mother, to a cheerful boy who enjoyed playdates, overnights with friends, and sleeping in his own bed. Dad was able to travel without wiping his son's tears. And Mom reported: "Enzo is happy and good."

Troubleshooting Tips

She's Not Belly Breathing: The stress of learning something new can make it hard for some kids to "get" the Balloon Breath, regardless of age. If your child is sucking in her belly or breathing into her chest, have her lie on her back. Then put something light on her stomach—a plush toy or a paperback book—and make it a game. See if she can make the object rise and fall with her breathing. Once she gets it, have her practice lying down until it feels natural, then have her try sitting or standing. Be patient. It may take some time, but the results are worth the wait.

He Fell Asleep: It's normal for people to fall asleep when they're learning to relax. If your child dozes off, let him be, but stay with him so he doesn't awaken alone. Then bring him back slowly and praise him for really relaxing! Clearly, he needed the rest. Just pick up again another day.

Tool 2. Discovering Your Special Place

There are private places within your child's inner world where he can work out problems or take mini-vacations from the stresses of life, where he can relax, regroup, or just hang out in a healthy way. Kids do this all the time when they play make-believe or daydream in class; they take themselves somewhere "else," to places and circumstances that are exciting and personal to them. This Tool redirects that natural "flight of fancy" into a path for self-care. While the Balloon Breath is the way in, the Special Place is a kind of stage for more imagination work, a calm inner environment where your child can face life's challenges. A springboard to some of the other Tools, it is also a profound skill on its own. Having a private sanctuary where you feel safe, loved, and appreciated is incredibly healing.

Use the following script to guide your child toward whatever Special Place he would like to create. He might find himself in a garden, a castle, a cave, or outer space. One child discovered "a room that can turn into anything"; another made frequent visits to the "Land of Far." It doesn't matter where yours goes or what he creates, as long as he feels protected. Once he finds safety inside, he is more likely to feel it outside, and he'll be more adaptable to challenges and change.

To introduce this Tool, say, "Let's take some time to find a place to relax." Or "Let's take a little vacation." Or simply present it as a game. Start with the Balloon Breath, then use this script to invite your child into a gentle inner journey. Combining the Balloon Breath and a Special Place is an excellent start for most situations.

SAMPLE SCRIPT Discovering Your Special Place

"Imagine yourself walking on a beautiful path. You might hear the sweet song of birds in the distance, feel soft grass under your feet, or brush past fragrant flowers along the way.

"In front of you is a carved wooden door with all your favorite colors. It has your name on it. Open it and step through. Good.

"Notice if you're indoors or out. You might be in a cozy room, a large, open meadow with trees and flowers, or somewhere else wonderful. You decide.

"This is your Special Place, where you can feel good about yourself. You deserve a peaceful place of your own. Here you are safe. You can play, study, rest, talk with whomever you wish, or do absolutely nothing.

"Surround yourself with everything and everyone that brings you joy. Invite people or animals you'd like to be with you. Whenever anyone walks through the door, they love and accept you just the way you are.

"If you've decided to be on your own, you can enjoy that, too. Let your imagination have a grand time. All this is for you. Remember who you really are: unique and important to this planet."

[Note: Close this imagery here or continue onto another Tool.

To end now, say: "When you're ready, come back here feeling refreshed and open your eyes."

To end at bedtime, say: "Now breathe deeply and allow yourself to fall asleep naturally."]

Practice Notes and Variations

Take the Lead: It can take time for kids to learn to go to their Special Place alone. Use this script, or your own adaptation, until you're sure your child knows the way. But don't let that stop you from teaching the other Tools. Just blend this script into the next.

Solo Travel: Once your child can find his own way, simply say, "Take some time to go to your Special Place, and let me know when you're there." He can lift a finger or nod his head—these small movements won't break his reverie. Continue when he's ready.

The Talking Tour: You may want to talk little kids to their Special Place, offering suggestions and eliciting feedback as you go. For instance, after your child imagines "stepping through" the door, ask what it looks like. Let her answer guide your next question. Give her cues and suggestions to spark her imagination. The conversation will keep her focused and connected.

Save Your Stories for Last: It's tempting to lead by example and tell her about your own Special Place, especially if you've been playing with the Tools on your own. But it's best to let her find her own spot, or to coach her with gentle suggestions. If you reveal first, she might just copy you or judge her own imaginings. Save your stories until she discovers her own space and shares it with you. Once she feels pleased and confident in her inner world, she will delight in learning about yours.

How Kids Use It

Five-year-old Candie felt isolated because she was more advanced than her kindergarten classmates. Reading at second grade level and performing two-digit addition and subtraction, she felt awkward with friends. She went to her Special Place to feel better about herself. "The way to get there is you climb on the clouds and hop from cloud to cloud," she said. "Birds fly all over. Mostly they know when I'm coming. Here I feel accepted." Retreating to her Special Place gave Candie the respite she needed. She came back ready to play with her peers.

Troubleshooting Tips

Nothing Comes: Don't let imagination become another source of pressure and disappointment for you or your child. Sometimes images take time to surface. Be patient. Perhaps your child is anxious or can't relax; hang out for a while. Give it time. Still nothing? Offer a little help. Take him on a Talking Tour (page 27) or prompt him with suggestions from his life: a family vacation spot, the setting of a favorite book, anywhere you've known him to be happy. Remind him that there is no right or perfect answer, and he can change places anytime.

She's Not Visual: Imagination is not only about "seeing"; it takes many forms. If your child isn't visually driven, try engaging her emotions and her other senses. What does it feel like to be there? Is she calm? Happy? What sounds are around her? Are there birds? A stream? Can she smell anything? Touch anything? The imagination is a room with many doors; one will open for her.

Stories Don't Compute: Kids' inner pictures can change within the same journey. Your child's Special Place might start out at the beach and end up in Alaska; a staircase may turn into an elevator or slide on the way down. It's all fine. The images don't have to be logical; they just need to make sense to him.

Nice Turns Ugly: What if you take your child on a soothing journey and horror images appear? It sometimes happens. When a child is relaxed, defenses drop; he may go to where upsetting images or thoughts hide. This can actually be helpful. After all, darkness exists; now's your chance to address it. He might even discover hidden resources. After one relaxation exercise, a nine-year-old boy drew a shark-infested ocean. Someone was about to be eaten. I nonchalantly asked, "Can anything help that poor guy?" "Oh yeah," the boy replied. "We could throw him this life preserver." Whenever you begin an imagination journey, remind him that if anything feels uncomfortable, he can toss it out and refocus on his breathing, or he can tell you and, together, you'll resolve it.

Tool 3. Meeting a Wise Animal Friend

Almost all children respond to animals, whether as pets, stuffed toys, wild creatures, or animated characters. An Animal Friend is an imaginary, loving protector who has a child's best interest at heart, and helps him access inner wisdom. Animal Friends offer unique perspectives. For instance, birds see from above, fish may swim under "emotional" waters, insects get the details, and dogs sniff out what humans can't see. They also represent instinct over logic; some problems require intuitive solutions. It's often more effective to ask an Animal Friend for advice than to reason through a problem. Of course, none of this is apparent to children. They just know they have an imaginary buddy they can rely on for wise help and support. And that's all they need to know.

Animal Friends can be fantasy creatures, real family companions, wild animals, or a combination. One girl was visited by a "dog-chicken"; another boy imagined a rainbow lizard. The possibilities are limitless. It's also common for kids to call up animals who mirror their feelings. A frightened child might encounter a nervous deer or a scared bunny. These fearful critters have just the understanding he needs to address his fear.

Though Animal Friends can't always remove problems, they do relieve your child's suffering. One seven-year-old boy's power animals, a pride of lions, stood guard around his hospital bed to keep him safe and give him the courage to face a frightening medical procedure.

Big kids and little ones alike resonate with Animal Friends. You can introduce this Tool with a question: "Have we gotten you an Animal Friend yet?" Or as a new game: "Let's find you an Animal Friend!" Or move into it without fanfare, directly from your child's Special Place.

SAMPLE SCRIPT   Meeting Your Animal Friend

"Take some time to focus on your Balloon Breath. Very nice.

"Remember your Special Place and let yourself go there . . . down your path . . . open the door and step inside. Get comfortable.

"When you're ready, ask for a wise and loving Animal Friend to arrive, one who wants the best for you. It may be an animal you know, one you've heard of, one that was once in your life, or even one you make up. Be surprised at who appears. Your Animal Friend is here to guide, protect, and help you with any concerns.

"When you're ready, tell your Animal Friend all about your problem. Ask for help: 'What do I need to know—or do—so I don't have to suffer with this?'

"What does your Animal Friend say?

"Ask questions to better understand your Friend's advice. Take all the time you need.

"When you're ready, focus on your breathing again. Notice how your feet and hands feel. Come back here, and slowly open your eyes."

....

Practice Notes and Variations

Pets and Preschoolers: Small children tend to imagine the animals they know: a family or friend's pet, critters they've seen in picture books, their own stuffed animals. These are great places to start. Try jogging your child's memory with pictures, reminders, or more specific questions: "Close your eyes and imagine what Fido or Kitty wants to tell you."

Trust His Imagination: The Animal Friends who arrive may not always make sense to parents. You may expect your nervous child to call in a brave Bear, but a timid Turtle shows up instead. Or your angry preteen encounters an equally angry Python. It's not uncommon. Children often seek understanding before solutions; they may reach for guides who can relate to them where they are. Greet each imagined friend and listen for its wisdom.

Welcome the Whole Team: Most kids meet one Animal Friend at a time, while some spontaneously encounter several at once, like the girl who discovered five swans in her healing pond. It all depends on the problem at hand and that child's need in that moment. Your child may have one Animal Friend for months, a different one each time, or a slew of animal buddies who arrive together. Just accept whoever shows up and help him discover how they can assist. You can also take the lead on this. If one Animal Friend isn't enough, ask who else is nearby. Sometimes a team makes all the difference.

How Kids Use It

Ten-year-old Ruth was an emotional girl who had trouble handling change. Vacations were hard because they created a departure from her comforting routines. Since she loved animals, we used a lot of Animal Friends in our work together. When a long summer break loomed, it was natural to call in a strong support team. I suggested she imagine animals in all directions: front, back, left, right, above, and below. There is a Native American tradition that uses these directions to call in power animals.[3] I adapted the idea for Ruth, and she jumped right in.

Sugar, a honey-colored Horse, appeared in front. He would stick up for Ruth if someone hurt her feelings. Snow-white Lambie had her back and lifted stress from it. When Ruth asked for extra help, Lambie suggested ways to reduce pressure, like tackling her summer reading list early and journaling her feelings. Red Fox, on her left, encouraged her to assert herself. Black Bird, on her right, offered white pellets of *Courage* to reduce anxiety in new places. Unicorn, below, reminded her to prepare for schoolwork in the fall. And Flying Piggy kept watch above to help with "anything else." With this kind of backup, Ruth had an easier summer.

Troubleshooting Tips

Nothing Comes: Always give your child the time and space to explore his own imagination. Sometimes, when nothing seems to come, it's the sign of a thoughtful mind feeling its way into something new. Wait a few minutes more and see how he responds. If he's still drawing a blank, offer suggestions of your own: the zebra at the zoo, a horse from a recent storybook, a neighbor's pet, any animal you know he has met, enjoyed, or read about. You don't even have to pick well. If he thinks your idea is silly, it may ignite some ideas of his own.

Scary Bears Arrive: Sometimes, if a child is stressed, a frightening animal may show up. But even scary guides offer wisdom and insight. Together, you can discover what this wild thing needs to calm down and feel better. First, create a sense of protection for her. Offer to put yourself on the scene or call another Animal Friend to the rescue. Or suggest that a gate or a fence appear between them. Whatever makes her feel safe enough to address the scary beast. Then ask what she wants to say to it. For example: "Go away." "Why are you acting up?" "How come you're being so mean?"

This can be a wonderful opportunity for discovery and healing. Fearsome images may be the hurt, dark parts of a child, trying to get attention. However, remind her that she can also make it simply go away and request that a nicer animal appear. She has the power to change any picture in her head, just like she changes TV channels. And she should always signal if she gets uncomfortable.

Tool 4. Encountering a Personal Wizard

We have a universal fascination with wizards and the idea that someone can wave a wand to make things right. Indeed, such magical beings are profound archetypes; they exist in all cultures and have endured in our stories and dreams since ancient times. Sometimes Animal Friends are not powerful enough. Kids may need or want real magic. That's when we bring in a Personal Wizard, a mentor and magical teacher in human form. When your child calls on a Wizard, she is supported by a collective imagination as old as the first fairytale and as new as the latest fantasy film. Wizards bring a different level of wisdom: human but extraordinary. Your child's Personal

Wizard will help her realize her own extra power to stretch and solve problems, while the charm of the magical can motivate her to take new risks.

Introduce this Tool with a conversation: "Today we'll learn to talk to Wizards. What do you know about them?" Use the script below and enjoy the surprise of who shows up.

SAMPLE SCRIPT

Encountering Your Personal Wizard

"Allow your eyes to gently close. Be aware of your breathing and follow it down your path to your Special Place. Take your time and let me know when you get there. Fine.

"Waiting for you is your own Wizard, ancient and all-knowing, coming to you from another realm. Because right now—today [and with this problem]—nothing less than magic will do.

"What does your Wizard look like? What clothing is he or she wearing? Which shoes and hat? Does she carry a wand?

"Notice everything, even how your Wizards smells, if he smiles, what he says to you.

"This wise and wonderful Wizard is here to be your Master Guide, as you face any problem. He will help you solve it with confidence and comfort.

"What magic does your Wizard perform to help you?

"Now imagine that your Wizard has a book called *All Information for All Time* and that it has the answers for any concern in the world.

"When your Wizard opens the book, what instructions help with your situation? What do you need to know or do?

"Listen to your Wizard's advice. Ask him to explain what you don't understand.

"When you're ready, take a deep Balloon Breath and bring your attention to your Heart. Slowly open your eyes."

Practice Notes and Variations

A Whole World of Wizards: Many Wizards show up in traditional garb—royal blue gowns and tall pointed caps decorated with stars. They are old, with long white beards. Yet today's Wizards can also come in all shapes and sizes. They may be young females or angels, mermaids, witches, or other mythical beings. These fulfill the same function as traditional Wizards. So can real people like a beloved grandparent who has died, or Albert Einstein, who showed up as one child's Math Wiz.

Call in a Specialist: Your child may have one Wizard or many. Some kids discover an All-Purpose Wizard, as well as "specialists" like a Confidence or Spelling Wizard. Some even have cool names like the Prince of Positive Thinking. To find one, just ask. Is your child having trouble with science? Suggest calling in a Science Wizard. Is her self-esteem low? Someone who can help her feel better about herself is in order. Observe her individual needs and guide her in that direction.

Mapping the Wizard World: Wizards, as magical creatures, have access to any astonishing place that you or your child can imagine. This makes them indispensable when more information is needed. I often invent useful, magical realms like the "Hall of Knowledge," which houses the book *All Information for All Time*, or the "Great Wise Room," where any question can be answered. Use these, or create your own corners of the Wizard world. Once a child can picture a place of limitless possibility, his imagination is free to offer unexpected answers.

The Magical Self: Sometimes your child may need help of an even more personal nature. Perhaps she needs to picture a healthy future or to understand a past hurt, maybe she's ready to rely more on her "own" wisdom than on an Animal Friend or Wizard, or she just needs one more perspective. Propose she consult herself . . . her *older* self, a year from now, with the problem solved; her *grown-up* self, successful and brave, from twenty years in the future; her *younger* self, the child who is still waiting to be healed and speaks her early need; or her *wisest* self, who knows more than she does. By talking to herself across time, she becomes her own magical being, offering an even deeper layer of personal wisdom.

How Kids Use It

Henry had gone to an alternative school for the first few years of his education. The kids there learned at their own pace, and social (not academic) development was emphasized. He'd never taken a test until he transferred to public school at nine. Almost two years later, he found himself in the fifth grade with only a third grader's grasp of multiplication. The Tool that worked best for him was Wizard Wisdom. Relaxed in his Special Place, Henry met Joe, the Math Wizard. He wore a trendy blue outfit with pointy red shoes and carried a star wand. Math Wizards were quite old, Henry explained. They ranged from 150 to 600 years, but his was on the younger side. Wizard Joe used multicolored flash cards to practice times tables, and sprinkled magic dust to help Harry remember them. He also directed him to a nearby apple tree. Every time Henry imagined eating a luscious ripe apple, he would get smarter. "Do a lot of Balloon Breaths," Joe advised before he left. "Stay calm at school, and call me if you need me."

Troubleshooting Tips

Nothing Comes: Wizards, at heart, are wise guides in human form. So if your child feels unable to locate a personal Wizard, perhaps that's because another type of wise or mythical being is waiting in the wings. If that doesn't work, and the call for a Wizard remains unanswered, stay positive and explain to your child that Wizards reveal themselves when they are really, really required. Maybe he doesn't need one yet, or his Animal Friends are doing a great job right now. Reassure him that when he does need a Wizard, one will surely show up.

Tool 5. Receiving Gifts from Inner Guides

Once your child is allied with an Animal Friend or Personal Wizard, he can ask for and receive Gifts from them. Gifts are much more than nice presents; they provide children with unique ways to receive power and assistance. They come in many forms: objects, thoughts, pictures, and ideas. They are often symbolic, metaphors for exactly what your child needs to cope with his dilemma. For instance, one lonely ten-year-old received a rose quartz heart to heal the sadness of her friend moving away: "I squeeze it tight, and there's no more loneliness." And a six-year-old's Wizard gave him a Ball of *Focus* to help concentrate at school.

The purpose of some Gifts can be obvious—like the child who received a flame to melt a "frozen heart"—or they may require further explanation by their Animal Friend or Wizard. Sometimes Gifts aren't given as much as discovered. They may be hidden or buried. An Animal Friend may help dig them up, or a Wizard might perform magic to make them stronger. The real giver, of course, is your child's own knowing. But the power of receiving the perfect Gift at the perfect moment cannot be overestimated. To receive Gifts, if they're not spontaneously offered, simply ask, "What Gift will help me right now?"

Receiving Gifts

"Focus on slow breathing and take yourself to your Special Place.

"When you are settled, ask for your guides—an Animal Friend or Wizard. Be patient. The right helper will come.

"Greet whoever shows up. Tell your guide your concerns and ask for something to help you in your life right now.

"Notice what Gift is offered. It may be a thought, a word, or something you can see or feel. It will guide you in your situation and show you how to overcome your problem.

"Ask questions about your Gift to understand its usefulness. Take all the time you need.

"When you are ready, focus on your Balloon Breath again, notice how you feel, and slowly open your eyes."

Practice Notes and Variations

Open or Shut? Sometimes a child receives a Gift, beautifully wrapped in shiny paper and a bow, but he doesn't want to open it. He's enjoying looking at the package so much, he just wants to keep gazing for a while. It's like seeing all his gifts together during holiday season. That's okay. He'll open his Gift when he's ready.

Many Gifts: It's perfectly fine if your child receives an abundance of Gifts—they'll be more ideas for solving his dilemma. Each Gift will offer another aspect of the solution. Sometimes I encourage receiving several Gifts as a child's story unfolds. Whatever seems right in the moment. Trust yourself.

How Kids Use It

Eight-year-old Elijah was a cautious, gentle soul whose world collapsed when older boys hid his clothes at a school campout. The initial humiliation quickly developed into anxiety. Quietly falling apart, he started sleeping badly and resisted solo activities. A Gift of *Legos* from his Wizard let him, literally, put things right. "I am the pieces," Elijah explained. "When I put myself together, I get stronger." He imagined going to Lego Land, where he took great satisfaction in building all kinds of structures. He even became a Lego truck and gave tours of the park. Without his realizing it, this imagination play seemed to restore his confidence. And piece by piece, his real-world interactions got sturdier, too.

Troubleshooting Tips

Nothing Comes: If your child asks for a Gift and nothing comes, or you ask about a Gift, only to be met with a blank stare or an "I don't know," then let it be for the moment. This takes practice. Sometimes children get nervous or tired, try to do the "right" thing, or just think too much. In my *Discovering Your Special Place* CD, I tell children to imagine that there is a Gift waiting in their imaginary Special Place and it will remind them how unique they are. But when I talk to them afterward, I find many don't notice one. I just tell them the Gift will still be there when they are ready. Reassure your child that anything he can't imagine now will come to him in time.

Confusing Gifts Appear: Sometimes children imagine Gifts whose meaning or use is unclear to them. This is when it helps to step in and be a little directive. Have your child ask an Animal Friend what the Gift is for, or suggest that her Wizard has special glasses that will let her see the instructions. Don't be afraid to use your imagination to help her unravel the puzzle. And trust that each Gift appears for a reason, even if it takes some footwork to find it.

Tool 6. Checking In with Heart and Belly

"Listen to your heart," people often say, or "What's your gut feeling?" It's a way to ask about intuition, a knowing that is different, maybe deeper, than logic. And it's good advice. The Belly and Heart have their own intelligence. Neuroscience has shown that certain "brain" chemicals—*neuropeptides*, which communicate with other parts of our bodies—don't live only in the brain; they also reside in our intestinal tract. This suggests a second "Belly Brain" for emotions.[4] Other research suggests that the heart has its own intelligence and communication system.[5] It's as if we have several brains in our bodies and each has something to offer.

Consider the heart transplant patient who develops a craving for the same ice cream as the donor, or a similar taste in music. Researchers in this area suggest a possible transfer of *cellular memory* from the donor's heart to the recipient's, as if the heart carries its own mini-brain.[6]

Checking in with Heart and Belly connects your child to his wisdom and develops his intuition—his ability to see, as some teachers say, "into the dark with the eyes of the heart."[7] The goal is not to forget the head, but to integrate Heart, Belly, and Mind in a way that steers your child to his personal truth.

Introduce this Tool with a few words about where we keep intuition: "You have so much knowledge in your brain, but your heart has wisdom for you, too. So does your belly. Let's focus on that and see what they have to say."

Heart and Belly Wisdom doesn't require a visit to a Special Place, although it's a nice start. Relaxing with the Balloon Breath is preparation enough.

Checking In with Heart and Belly

"Close your eyes gently and pay attention to your breathing. Notice the air going in your nose and traveling down to your belly. Breathe out just as slowly.

"Now bring your attention to your Heart in the middle of your chest. Imagine it beating, filled to the top with love and wisdom.

"Ask your Heart what message it has for you. What's important for you to know today? You can even have a conversation with it.

"If you haven't spoken to your Heart for a while, it may be shy. Practice waiting. It will tell you what you need to know.

"Listen closely to Heart's message. Take its words deep inside and thank it.

"Now move your attention to your Belly—where your gut feelings live. Let it speak to you, too.

"What is Belly's wisdom for today? Is it the same as Heart's? Or does Belly say something very different?

"Tell your Belly and Heart about any concerns you have. Ask for advice.

"If Heart and Belly suggest two different solutions, encourage them to talk to each other. What does Belly need Heart to know? What does Heart say? How can they work together?

"When you're ready, tell Heart and Belly you'll be back soon, maybe even tomorrow. Say good-bye and return your attention here."

Practice Notes and Variations

The Tender Touch: Talking and listening to the Heart and Belly is a new concept for children. One way to make it real is to have your child put his hand over his heart while he imagines the inner conversation. Not only does this make the connection more concrete, but it's physically comforting. The same is true for the belly. The connection may feel more intimate when he offers his tummy a tender touch.

Check In Often: Like the Balloon Breath, this is a great daily practice. When it feels natural, encourage your child to take a few minutes each morning to "check in" with his Heart and Belly after settling himself with his slow breathing. Once he hears that day's message, he can apply its wisdom to all his interactions.

How Kids Use It

Nine-year-old Opal felt so guilty about her misbehavior at school that her tummy ached. But she didn't know how to change her bullying ways. I suggested she go straight to her Heart and Belly and ask them for advice. Heart took on her mother's loving voice: "I believe in you and know you can make better choices." Belly volunteered to repair mistakes. Both promised to lead her to other options; all she had to do was check in with them daily. All on her own, she imagined them cheering her up, singing, "Once glad, stay glad. Once sad, don't stay sad. Get on the road to Happy Town!" Opal learned to start her day by checking in with Heart and Belly Wisdom, just a quick sixty seconds. Her behavior slowly improved, her tummyaches left, and she felt good about taking care of herself in such a positive, powerful way.

Troubleshooting Tips

Nothing Comes: Sometimes a child asks for Heart or Belly advice, only to be met with silence. This is not unusual. These are new lines of communication and awareness; they take time to nurture. "Your

Heart (or Belly) is just not used to talking to you," I tell children. "It may be a little bashful and want to know you're serious about listening to it. It might take a little time, but keep trying. Just check in every day. Heart and Belly will come around."

Tool 7. Talking to Toes and Other Body Parts

Just as Heart and Belly have their wisdom, so does the body at large. We seem to stash feelings and symptoms in almost every part of it, with our body becoming a repository for lots of hidden information. This Tool invites your child to look inside and see what she can learn from her body; it provides information about emotions and physical symptoms that you might not access with other Tools. Talking to Body Parts can reveal the fears and worries that turn tension into physical pain; it also makes elusive feelings concrete so that your child can work with them in creative and healing ways.

Of course, while pain and muscle spasms are obvious, there is no map or descriptions for feelings. *Worry* might be in the belly, *Courage* in the chest, and *Sadness* in the eyes. But Worry could just as easily live in hands and Courage in legs. Your child's discoveries will be as unique as she is.

With the script as a guide, she will learn to converse with her emotions and body parts—and also among them—to find solutions to her concerns. *Confidence* might talk to a tummyache or *Anger* might speak for a headache.

The first time you try this Tool, work with two to four simple feelings, half positive (love, calm, brave) and half negative (angry, sad, scared). Let your child lead the way with whatever feelings are "up" for her in the moment.

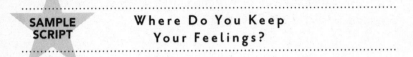

Where Do You Keep Your Feelings?

"Use your Balloon Breath to relax. We're going to be detectives and find out where your feelings live. All of them are important and have valuable information for you. Close your eyes and picture searching inside your body.

"Let's start with some good ones. Where does *Happiness* hang out? *Love? Calm? Brave?* What shape do they have? What color?

"Now let's find some uncomfortable feelings. Where do you keep *Angry* feelings? *Sad? Worry?* What do they look like?

"Pick one good and one not-so-good feeling. See what each has to say. What does Calm want to tell Anger? What does Brave say to Worry? Listen to them with kindness. It can be tough to talk about true feelings.

"How can they live together peacefully and help each other? What suggestions do they have? Good.

"Each time we do this, we'll visit more feelings.

"That's enough for today. Remember what you've learned and slowly come back."

Practice Notes and Variations

Check In . . . Whenever You Want: This is another good, anytime Tool. Learning to address feelings directly can often disable the aches and pains that speak up instead. Like Checking In with Heart and Belly, this Tool takes little preparation. Just start with a few minutes of the Balloon Breath, and go right in.

Play Both Sides: It's valuable to identify and express negative feelings, yet it's just as important to offer hope and change. This Tool assumes that each negative feeling has a healthy partner that lives somewhere in your child—*Fear* and *Courage*, *Sad* and *Happy*—even if it's a tiny spec that can be expanded.

Body Time: Use this Tool whenever you need to understand or address the feelings behind a symptom or behavior, such as worry under a stomachache or jealousy behind a sibling squabble. It's also useful when emotions are obvious and overwhelming, like hurt and anger at being left out of schoolyard games. Once your child can describe a negative feeling in her body, you can help her discover the inner antidote.

Tiny Talk: Most little kids are comfortable imagining the shape or location of their feelings, but they can get lost in the language. Make sure to choose feeling words that your child understands. If *Angry* is unfamiliar, try *Mad* or *Upset*.

Pain Talks, Too: Physical symptoms, like headaches, stomachaches, bad backs, and nervous tics, respond well to this Tool. By adapting the script for a conversation with pain or real body parts, your child can discover what his sore spots look like, what they have to say, and what they need to stop hurting.

How Kids Use It

At ten, Thomas was stoic. He never shed tears and wouldn't admit defeat, but inside he worried. His wise Heart and Belly echoed my encouragement to express his feelings, but he wasn't sure how. So Thomas began to check in with different emotions; he discovered where they lived in his body and what messages they had for him. *Stress* was in his head. It had a lot to say: "I have to do my homework! Am I ever going to graduate middle school? Am I ever going to be a real artist? What about the war?" With such pressure, no wonder Thomas felt overwhelmed.

He turned to *Calmness* (in his arms) to see how to handle Stress. "Just do your homework," *Calm* said. "Don't worry too much; it's all right to have fun." Then *Fear*, wiggly in his legs, came forth with: "I might be a bad person. Everyone around me is bad." *Sad* eyes chimed in, "I feel like a glass breaking." *Love* in his chest became the antidote for disturbing feelings. "You've done some good things," it assured him, "and there is good in the world. Try to love something in everything and everybody." By the time this conversation ended, Thomas felt hopeful about a better future.

Troubleshooting Tips

Nothing Comes: Some kids have a hard time locating feelings in their body. It's more of a leap than picturing a Special Place or talking to an Animal Friend. If your child seems stuck, give her a little extra time—in case she's feeling her way into it—and then offer some examples. You could say, "Sometimes when we're sad, we feel it in our Heart, or in our eyes when we cry. Some people feel anger in their fists or feet because they want to punch or kick someone. Do you keep your anger in your fists or feet?" A "wrong" suggestion on your part might still help her find what's real for her.

He's Not Visual: Again, imagery isn't only about visual pictures. Your child may think an image, smell, feel, taste, or hear it. In one training workshop, a therapist said he didn't "do" movies in his head, but he heard music. His stress was a loud concerto; love was a passionate opera. Perhaps your child's *Worry* is sticky or sounds like a kitten crying; maybe *Happiness* smells like wet dirt or tastes like chocolate. There are many ways for your child to create vivid "pictures" of his feelings. Be open to however your child receives creative insight. Stay flexible.

There's No Other Side: It's rare, but occasionally a child is unable to locate an antidote feeling. Maybe the bad feelings are too big, or she doesn't believe good ones are possible. When that happens, I use memory as a trigger. "How do you feel when you get presents for your birthday?" I ask a child who's trying to find *Happy*. Once she recalls that moment and its Happiness, we can investigate where that emotion lives in her body. You know the moments your child has experienced *Calm*, *Brave*, and other good feelings. You can use that knowledge to help him remember, and reimagine, them now.

The Feelings Keep Moving: Feelings may change location and shape during imagery, even within the same session. For instance, *Fear* may start out in your child's chest and, by the end of the time together, reside in her belly. *Anger* may move from her head to her hands. Don't worry. This is not about consistency but awareness. What matters is that she is able to notice her feelings, locate them in her "body/mind," and remain true to herself in the moment.

Tool 8. Using Color for Healing

Color is a powerful tool for transforming pain, whether it's physical, emotional, or even a spiritual longing to connect. Almost everyone can relate feelings to colors. Think about how some people are "green with envy," while others just "feel blue." It's a shorthand that lets us see what can't be seen and explain it to others.

Associations are unique to each individual. Anger can be "roaring red" for one person and "raging black" for another—or different for the same person on different days. The specifics don't matter; it's the way color expresses our feelings and captures our imaginations that's important.

Your child can use Color to reduce physical pain and shift emotions. Striking colors may be associated with headaches and stomachaches. One child's tummy felt like green gunk; she used gold *Love* from her Heart to clean it out. Another's headache was fire engine red; he cooled it with blue ice. The same occurs with emotions. Color can transform negative feelings—purple *Courage* calming orange *Fear*—and it can pump up the volume on good feelings such as *Joy* and *Love*. Once your child discovers where feelings reside in his body and what they look like (Tool 7), he can add Color to that information for healing.

As you begin, identify the colors of one negative feeling and two positive ones, like blue *Brave* and green *Confidence* facing gray *Fear*. They may be the same ones from the last Tool, or they may be new. What happens when we breathe the color of *Calm* into *Anger*, for instance? What about the color of *Love*? Which works better? Use the sample script to play with possibilities. Experiment. You don't know what will happen until it does.

SAMPLE SCRIPT   Use Color for Healing

"Let's experiment with color. Imagine your *Happy* feelings—what color are they? What color is *Excitement*? Or *Peace*? Take your time . . .

"Now focus on today's *Sad* or *Bad* feelings. What color are they?

"Which color will you use to calm those bad feelings? Ask inside and see what pops up.

"Whatever color you picked, breathe it slowly and gently into the *Sad* or *Bad* feelings. Keep breathing until you fill up that whole area.

"Now take that good color and fill your whole body with it, from the top of your head to the tip of your toes. Notice what happens.

"Feel that color swirling all through your body, filling every inch of you with good feelings. Remember what this feels like. Enjoy it for a bit.

"When you're ready, take a deep breath and come back here, feeling centered and refreshed."

Practice Notes and Variations

Two Against One: It's useful to work colors and feelings in sets of three: two positive and one negative. If one doesn't work, the other might. Your child can try to blend them and see what happens.

Healing White: Sometimes a child will reach for color and nothing comes, or there are too many to choose from and he gets confused. When in doubt, try white, which contains all the colors of the spectrum. Have him imagine it as a color or light pouring through his body, turning into whatever he needs at the time.

How Kids Use It

Helena, a sweet seven-year-old, was referred by her pediatrician for chronic stomachaches. Her parents were on the verge of an unspoken divorce, and her little body suffered from their constant arguments. She described her pain as a thunderous cloud of smoke. When she asked her stomach what color might make her feel better, a swirling rainbow appeared. By breathing in this multicolored healing light, Helena reduced her pain. She also learned to use Color to protect her Heart. Pure white light transformed her black misery, becoming a kaleidoscope of colors to shield her from parental disputes. The first time she did this, Helena was delighted. It was, she said, "Like I was in the middle of the sun with golden lightbulbs going through my body."

Troubleshooting Tips

Blue Won't Stay Blue: Like the location and shape of feelings (page 47), your child may shift the color of things. *Sorrow* may be brown one moment and blue the next. *Happy* may switch from red to yellow. Again, there is no cause for concern. As long as he is expressing his feelings, he is in the process of learning and healing.

Tool 9. Tapping Into Energy

When words and images are insufficient, a loving touch can do wonders to restore calm and well-being. Healing energy practices have existed across many cultures since time immemorial. Some involve hands-on massage and energetic touch while others employ good thoughts and prayers. Now science is confirming their effectiveness. Recent research with brain scans (fMRIs) showed that when energy healers sent "distant intention" (their desire to offer health and well-being) to subjects inside scanners, definite areas of the receiver's brain were activated, yet none of the recipients knew when these thoughts were being sent.[8] This study, which used a variety of techniques, from Japanese Reiki and Chinese Qi Gong to Peruvian shamanism, is an exciting look at the possible effects of healing energy.

Of course, you don't need to be a Reiki master or shaman to use energy with your child. Your love is powerful in and of itself; you can release it through your hands, eyes, and thoughts. By directing it with intention, you may effect tangible changes in your child's physical or emotional state. And you can teach her to do the same for herself.

Preparing to Tap Into Energy

Experience the feel of physical energy by simply rubbing your hands together quickly for about a minute, then letting them slowly part. Can you sense the invisible vibration between them? It might feel like a heaviness or magnetic pull. Play with it, moving your hands in and out slowly like an accordion. Or shape it into a ball, first big like a beach ball, then small like a tennis ball.

Simple Exercises

Healing Touch: You can use the loving energy you feel toward your child to reduce physical and emotional hurts. Focus on your Balloon Breath and imagine your Heart's love moving through your arms into your hands, filling them with a continuous flow of caring energy. Gently place your hands wherever your child experiences discomfort. Keep a neutral and loving state of mind. Think of this as an extension of "kissing the boo-boo" on a skinned knee. Be sure to wash your hands afterward, or imagine cleaning them with light, to avoid absorbing her uncomfortable feelings.

Healing Gaze: Gather the love in your Heart and send it into your eyes. Concentrate on sending loving energy as you gaze at your child.

Healing Thought: Imagine your child as healthy and happy and having overcome any challenges she may face. Send those positive thoughts to her whenever you can.

Energy Self-Care for Kids

Have your child imagine sending love from her Heart into her hands. Show her how to rub her hands together and separate them to feel the energy. Then have her place them on her tummy for several minutes. If it hurts, she may experience relief; if it doesn't, she might just feel warmth. It's a good Tool to practice when she's well, so that it's available if her Heart or body is sore.

Together, you can find fun ways to play with energy. It will increase the positive vibrations in both your bodies and your lives.

SAMPLE SCRIPT — Energy Self-Care for Kids

"Let's play with the energy and the good vibes around you.

"Imagine the *Love* that's in your Heart growing larger as you do your Balloon Breath. Each time you breathe, you spread your Love out more. Picture it growing so large that Love fills up your chest and moves down your arms into your hands.

"Feel it in your fingertips—it might be tingling. Or your hands might feel warmer as you send more Love to them. Can you feel how warm your hands are getting?

"Keep doing your Balloon Breaths, nice and slow.

"Now put your hands on your Belly and let them stay there awhile. How does it make your tummy feel?"

If there is any pain: "Imagine any pain leaving your body and disappearing harmlessly.

"Keep your healing hands there for as long as you like.

"When you're ready, lift your hands off your Belly and slowly open your eyes."

How Kids Use It

Four-year-old Win-Lee and his family had recently emigrated to the United States from Asia and spoke little English. He was put in preschool, where he acted out, hitting and kicking other children to get his way. He was also constantly moving and unable to concentrate at circle time. His teachers referred him to a Chinese-speaking psychologist who diagnosed him as hyperactive and recommended medication. But his parents didn't want to put such a young child on medicine. They didn't know where to turn, until a colleague referred them to me.

At our first meeting, Win-Lee's parents, their translator, and I watched as he ran through my office, touching everything. I spoke in a calm voice, without knowing how much he understood. Under such circumstances, and with his parents' agreement, energy work seemed the best option. After centering myself with deep breaths, I placed my hands on his low back and belly, sending him loving, peaceful thoughts. It calmed him immediately. He gravitated toward me and wanted to sit on my lap. We played together with blocks on the floor, and he stayed near me the whole session. This continued for several weeks and was the only intervention I made, but soon Win-Lee's behavior improved at school, and his teachers stopped complaining. Our simple energy work had balanced him.

Troubleshooting Tips

Nothing Comes: Some children may not "feel" anything initially—not when you place your hands on them or when they're learning energy self-care. That's understandable since energy work might be new to them. And many people—adults and children alike—feel little when they receive energy. Not to worry. Just trust that your love is reaching them. If your child doesn't feel anything in her *own* hands after using the script, then teach her Preparing to Tap Into Energy (page 51), just like you learned it. This playful exercise will give her a more direct experience of subtle vibrations.

It Feels Weird: A child may feel something but not know what to make of it. She might try to wash or shake off the sensation. No problem. As she becomes aware of these energy feelings, they'll become familiar friends. And she can learn to wash them away with water or thought when she's done.

Putting It All Together

Each of the Nine Tools is powerful medicine on its own, but the real magic comes when you mix and match them to fit your child's changing needs. The pictures he imagines will teach him to feel safe and secure in any circumstance, since his inner wisdom is the ultimate source of what to do. And you are the guide to releasing the knowledge that lies within.

CHAPTER 3

The Benefits of Artistic Expression

Keeping a journal with my writings and drawings makes me feel better.

—*Pearl, age seven*

Combining Imagery Tools with Music, Drawing, and Writing

★ Since the first drums and cave paintings, we humans have found creative ways to express ourselves. We play, sing, and revel in music. We draw, paint, and doodle. We capture thoughts and feelings on paper. And we share our creations with others. But the arts do more than communicate and entertain; they soothe our souls, clarify our thinking, and even soften our body's stress responses. Applied to the Nine Tools, music, drawing, and writing act like a booster pack, enhancing the healing that imagery inspires. In fact, when you add artistic expression, the richness of imagination becomes three-dimensional. Music deepens relaxation and concentration, while drawing and writing offer alternate ways "in" to the private mind. The ability to express on paper the truth of the heart and mind makes those images concrete and more powerful. Your child's artistic expression will also give you a clearer sense of his inner struggle, an insight that will help you guide him toward each next step.

Melodious Music

Soothing the Soul

The healing influence of music on health and behavior has been recognized since the writings of Aristotle and Plato.[1] In fact, in Greek mythology, Apollo was the god of music *and* medicine; a pairing that makes sense in light of modern research. Studies find that listening to soothing music reduces pain, anxiety, depression, and seizures. It also stabilizes irregular heartbeats and strengthens pulse and breathing. One study with premature infants discovered that music stimulates the brain's alpha waves, creating a feeling of calm[2]—something lullaby-singing mothers have known for centuries.

Music also facilitates learning. In young children, it helps build neural pathways that support the development of language, memory, and spatial intelligence (the ability to visualize the world accurately).[3] Indeed, IQ scores in spatial-temporal reasoning among college students increased after listening to just ten minutes of a Mozart sonata.[4] Another study found that music enrichment classes improved math and reading scores in public school children.[5]

Although researchers have tested a variety of styles and composers, few have received the scrutiny of Mozart, whose harmonies are recognized for stimulating the brain and relaxing the muscles.[6] "The Mozart Effect"[7] is a common term for the transformational influence Mozart's music has on health and well-being. In one study, a Spanish dairy farmer played Mozart to 700 heifers. The cows that were exposed to the music lined up quietly to be milked and produced up to six more liters a day than those who were not. Their milk also had higher levels of healthy fats and proteins and, they say, a sweeter taste.[8] If music can enhance milk production in cows, imagine what it can do for your child's imageries.

How to Use It

Create a Soundtrack: Playing gentle background music can strengthen the healing effect of imagery by accelerating relaxation and helping children stay peaceful throughout the journeys and conversations that follow. It's especially useful when you first teach the Tools. By practicing them with music, your child will connect the experience with a deeper tranquility, even when the music is gone. As you move forward, it may not always be practical or necessary to turn on the CD player—quick check-ins don't require it. But when you do have time for a longer "session," it's always good to have a selection of favorites to work with. Discover which music soothes your child and create your own playlist. Lyrics can be distracting, so look for instrumentals. I use a wide range of composers, including Steven Halpern, P. C. Davidoff, Mark Provost, Nawang Khechog, Constance Demby, Kevin Braheny, Georgia Kelly, Kitaro Ki, George Winston, and Paul Horn. Try one of these or start your own collection.

Understand the Music Zone: Sometimes when you take a child on a guided journey using music, you may lose him after a minute or two. He may be transported to a blissful, melodic spot. That's fine. He's simply dropping inside himself to a place of peace, where creativity develops and ideas emerge. He doesn't have to hear all your words; they'll be there next time. This deep rest gives him an important opportunity to rebalance.

Sound Off: Although not always melodic, the making of simple sounds is part of your child's internal music and can transform her state of being, either energizing or calming her. Too often kids release trapped energy or emotions by hitting or kicking, when sound is what's really required. Encourage your child to vocalize her feelings during imagination work. Maybe she wants to sing, growl, grunt, or roar. Discovering what her angry or sad parts sound like can be another helpful piece of the puzzle, not to mention a relief for your child.

Scribbles and Strokes

Drawing as Emotional Release

Like music, art has been used throughout history for healing. Studies show that it creates brain wave patterns that enhance the autonomic nervous system, hormonal balance, and brain neurotransmitters. During expressive art, the body's physiology shifts from stressed to serene.[9]

Art supports and reinforces imagery. Once your child has accessed his feelings through imagination, he can release them in a drawing. Because it's often easier to talk about pictures than about himself, drawing will allow your child to express difficult feelings or to disclose what he might not share verbally.

Drawing also increases your child's awareness of his inner world and creates a window onto that landscape. When I lead a child through imagery, I don't know what's going on in his mind until we talk. His drawings are a useful addition to our conversations, helping reveal that inner Self. They let me see, literally, the squiggly green *Anger* snaking up his leg, the purple *Happiness* in his arms, or the *Sad* Heart with the blue tears. We can then work with, or through, the picture. If he paints a monster about to eat him up, I might ask, "Oh, can anything help?" It's not that I want to take away his uncomfortable feelings prematurely, but I want to discover what resources he has. If he says, "I'll get a shovel and hit him over the head," his response tells me he's thinking in terms of taking action and has figured out at least one way to take care of himself. That's a good starting point for delving deeper into his fears. If he has no idea what to do, I'll offer a thought or two, like calling Mom or Dad for help or telling the monster to go away, and see if he goes for it. If he doesn't, we have even more work to do.

Similarly, your child's drawings can offer you more than just a picture of her feelings. They can launch conversations that reveal her thinking about the world around her, whether she can imagine solving her problems, and who or what might help her do that. And they provide opportunities for you to help her recognize support where she might not perceive it.

A child's artwork also gives him a way to remember and connect with his reveries and to track his own changes. One boy derived comfort creating a greeting card and putting it on his dresser so his recently deceased grandpa could see it from Heaven. And when an eight-year-old girl drew herself as a delightful princess, I knew how much her fragile self-image had grown, since her prior self-portraits had been as an unhappy gremlin.

How to Use It

Stock Up on Supplies: Although any pencil will do, I like to use a variety of crayons, pens, and markers. So many fun ones are available: fat, thin, smelly, sparkly, metallic, even markers that change as they write over another color. Your child's imagination is a vivid place; you'll want her pictures to reflect that.

Draw a Snapshot: Many kids benefit from identifying where their feelings are early in the process through their drawings. Help little ones by tracing their body on large sheets of paper and letting them fill in the "map." Older ones can design and complete their own.

Picture the Future: Artwork is also an effective starting point when you're working with clear end-goals, like getting a good night's sleep or reducing a fear. Have your child draw two pictures: one of how things are now, and one of how he'd like them to be. Seeing the current "mess" of his life in full color on paper and transforming it into an equally vivid picture of his goal is inspiring. Five-year-old April scribbled a mean purple face to show her present behavior and a happier smiling version of herself in pink, representing the kindness she wanted to attain. Kids often hang these pictures in their bedroom to remind them of their desired direction.

Show and Tell: Drawing the experience after an imagery journey is another valuable endeavor. The picture gives you both something to look at and discuss. It may indicate your next step. If the drawing illustrates a problem—say, a dangerous goblin or a fire at home—ask her what might solve the situation. If she doesn't know, offer a few suggestions. This gives her alternative resources. If she thinks nothing can help, then take that hopelessness as an opportunity to teach her that there are always solutions, even if we don't yet see them.

Accept Every Drawing: Some kids have a tough time committing their mental pictures to paper; they fear they won't measure up. Reassure your child that anything he creates will be fine, even if it has nothing to do with his imagery. Sometimes all that comes are strokes of bold color evolving out of a wonderful or terrible feeling that is finally set free on paper. Praise each one. They are the artifacts of your child's inner world.

Talk to the Image: Once your child has spilled his feelings on paper, he can converse with them. He might use his picture of *Fear* to ask what it needs to calm down, or tell it to leave. It's much easier to speak to feelings when they're outside, than when they're eating at his tummy.

Take Artistic Action: It's a great release when a child can draw her angry, hurt, or upset feelings, but pictures don't have to be static.

She can erase part of it, or draw over it in "healing" colors with a changeable marker—an immediate transformation that feels magical. She can even rip up or throw away the paper. These actions can offer a hurting child a sense of control and satisfaction.

Capture the Memory: The Special Places your child visits on her journey are personal healing sanctuaries. Hanging pictures of them somewhere private but visible will remind her that she can return whenever the need arises. Drawings of trusted Animal Friends and Wizards can help her remember that support is always near.

Taking Pencil to Paper

Writing for Healing

Diaries, letters, poems, songs, lists, and emails—we're always using words to reveal feelings and sort our thoughts. Something about them makes us feel better, and not just in mood. Researchers have found writing about things that affect us deeply favorably impacts our quality of life physically and emotionally. Emotional writing—whether to clear an upset or envision positive scenarios—lowers blood pressure, heart rate, and pain levels, and improves the immune system. It also reduces sleep disruption in cancer patients. It decreases depression and anxiety, as well, while promoting a more optimistic view of life.[10] And studies with elementary school kids found that regular journaling raises creativity and improves achievement. In fact, reading and math scores increased as much as 20 percent in one year.[11]

There are many ways children can use writing to enhance healing and problem solving. My two favorites are journaling and writing with the nondominant hand.

Keeping a Journal

Whether it's a pretty locked diary or a notebook covered in stickers, a journal is a great outlet for your child and a perfect complement to imagination work. Journals offer a safe and private place for her to express herself without judgment or failure. And while writing about upsets may sadden her briefly, the long-term results are worth it. A simple way to start is by writing a page upon waking or at night, just to clear her mind.[12] Younger children can dictate their feelings while you write them down. But even if frequent journaling doesn't appeal to her, she can still use the power of writing to enhance her imagination work.

Write After Imagery: This allows a child to explore her thoughts and feelings about the experience in a private, concentrated way. It also teaches her self-reflection and self-observation. Once she writes about her imagery, she can choose to share it with you or not. And since it's on paper, she can always show it to you later.

Write a Letter: Letters are a perfect way to communicate with an absent person or a feeling you want to engage. Writing an expressive (unmailed) letter to a challenging friend, a younger self, a grandparent who has passed, or even to physical pain can give your child an unexpected way to access information and create peace of mind.[13]

Writing with the Nondominant Hand

Like imagery, writing with the nondominant hand is associated with the right hemisphere of the brain and taps directly into intuition. I usually introduce this technique after a child has already mastered many of the imagery Tools, typically when he encounters a problem that his imagery can't solve, when he's more verbally driven, or once he has drawn a few pictures and can use more direct information. However, I reserve this process for slightly older kids, fourth grade and up; it's too difficult for younger ones who are still honing their normal writing skills.

It doesn't matter which hand you normally write with; when you switch to the other, you invite the unexpressed parts of your Self to speak.[14] For instance, when ten-year-old Shawn used his dominant hand to ask, "Why do I have so much stress when I'm at school?" he discovered he felt a lot of pressure that wasn't really there. "I'm putting it on myself," his nondominant hand told him. "I think my parents are pressuring me to do well, but they aren't." When he asked how to reduce his pressure, the other hand wrote, "Just relax and do your imagery every day." This is a fabulous way for a child to access repressed emotions and hidden wisdom.

Use Colors to Ask Hands: Have your child choose two pens or markers in whichever colors attract him, one color per hand. He should hold both of them in order to keep track of which color represents which hand. Now he can have a "conversation" between the two, using them to investigate issues on behalf of his logic and intuition. His logical dominant hand can interview his angry or sad feelings, or a younger or wiser older Self. It can even contact the healer within. We have a storehouse of natural chemicals in our brain that, when released, can relieve our suffering; the nondominant hand often holds a key to that medicine chest.

Whatever your child is exploring, begin with a question. "What would he like to ask?" If he doesn't know, offer several choices. For instance: "What does *Anger* want? Why is it here? What do I need to know about it?" If he's talking to a sad, younger self, he might ask, "How old are you? Why are you sad?" Or for the healer within, "Where is the button that turns off pain? What do I need to do?"

Have him pick one question, do three Balloon Breaths to calm himself, and start writing with the nondominant hand. Not thinking, but writing. This is not linear. If he can just go with it, he'll find that different thoughts pop into his mind when he uses each pen.

Take the Slow Road: Remember, talking between hands is slower than vocal conversations. He may feel impatient and silly at first because it's physically challenging, but it's also funny to see how odd the writing looks. And it produces information that may not otherwise surface.

Follow Whitney's Lead: Whitney was an extremely shy eleven-year-old who was just learning to communicate with herself this way. We were working on opening her up to what brought her joy. Her hand-to-hand interview is a great example of how this works.

Whitney's Dominant Hand (DH): Why don't you speak up?
Whitney's Nondominant Hand (ND): I don't know why.
DH: I want you to speak up.
ND: I don't think so.
DH: Let's just try a little bit. I won't get mad. I want to talk.
ND: Okay. I like to sing.
DH: Thank you. I like to sing, too. What else do you like to do?
ND: I like to dance.
DH: When would you like to dance?
ND: Next Thursday at 5 p.m.
DH: I will ask my mom to look into a class.
ND: Good.
DH: What else do you like to do?
ND: I like to write stuff.
DH: What kind of stuff do you like to write?
ND: Stories mostly, and plays.
DH: Would you like me to write more?

ND: Yes.

DH: What else do you like to do?

ND: I like to swim.

DH: I don't like to swim. How do we resolve this?

ND: We don't have to go.

DH: Would a bath be as good as swimming?

ND: Uh-hmm.

DH: How often?

ND: One to three mornings.

DH: Thank you. When would you want to talk again?

ND: Welcome. Not now.

DH: Is it okay if we talk every day or something?

ND: Yes.

Because Whitney was new to this, her questions and answers were short and simple. As she got comfortable, they became more fluid. She also seemed to contradict herself, but ambivalence is a natural part of life. Some part of her was curious about swimming; another was wary. These are the contradictions that nondominant writing negotiates well. This time the solution was a bath; next time she could invite herself into a real pool. All kinds of possibilities arise when a child establishes such communication with herself.

Music, drawing, and writing all boost the effectiveness of the Nine Tools. Background music opens a door to quicker and deeper relaxation, while drawing and writing are both ways for you and your child to gain more insight and to interact—tangibly—with elusive feelings and images. Together, they provide a foundation for healing many of the hurts and challenges children face—and their parents, too.

CHAPTER 4

Grown-Ups Need Tools, Too

My Heart said, "Love
yourself, all is well," and
my Belly said, "Eat joy
every day!"

—A mom

Tips for Less Stress and Better Parenting

★ Janice was truly stressed. Her three kids did nothing but bicker. Her neck was so tense it felt like wood. She was convinced that if only she were a better mother, her children would get along. Bonnie was frustrated and embarrassed that her ten-year-old son kept acting out at school. "I'm that mother," she complained, "the one who can't control her kid." Meanwhile, Ray knew he was being short-tempered at home. His estranged brother was in a coma, and his grief kept erupting as irritation toward his daughters. It hurt to see their cautious looks, but he didn't know how to calm himself.

Parenting, under the best circumstances, is a tough job. And that's before the natural stressors of life up the ante. You want to do your best, but sometimes it's impossible. All of us have been the impatient parent, the exhausted adult, the overworked partner. All of us are scrambling to be a good mom or dad. Some have had great role models; others haven't. Many of my clients say they're trying to avoid what their parents did. I tell them not to worry; they'll make other mistakes. That's just human. It not only takes a village to raise a child, it takes a lifetime.

With the first baby, a parent is born. Your experience is as young as your child, and you're both still growing. Meanwhile, you're doing the best you can in the moment. So be kind. Accept where you are. Practice self-forgiveness when you mess up. And don't be afraid to apologize to your kids if you need to. These actions will teach them valuable life lessons.

The same Nine Tools you are teaching your children offer you a path to calmer and better parenting. I give Good Health Homework to every parent who attends my workshops. "Pick three Tools," I tell them. "Start today, and email me in a week." I also teach my top ten list, "What Kids Most Want and Need from Their Parents." The results are as profound for adults as for kids.

Self-Care for Adults

As with your children, regular use of the Nine Tools can teach you to relax, develop your intuition, and trust your inner wisdom. Read through the Tools in Chapter 2 again, now with your own needs in mind. Where's your Special Place? What Gifts would you like? When did your Heart and Belly last have a conversation? How can your imagination address *your* life challenges?

It may feel silly at first. Animal Friends and Wizards aren't common fixtures of grown-up life, and parents are sometimes shy to use them. But so much adult suffering begins in childhood, and the Tools—because they are playful—are perfect for reaching that wounded kid inside.

Adults are often surprised and delighted when they discover how vibrant and healing their own imaginations can be. One mom received the Gift of a *Golden Voice* so she could make an important presentation in front of a large group. Another connected with Heart wisdom concerning a delicate situation between her son and her ex-husband. "Follow me, and you'll know what to do," her wise Heart told her.

This self-reassurance gave her the confidence to create a clear course of action. One dad received permission in his Special Place to share intense feelings, something that's still rare for men in our culture. "I went to a pool in an enclosed rocky space," he explained. "There by the pool was a box with *Tissues* written on it. The message was that it's all right to cry; it's not a weakness. It felt reassuring."

Whatever your personal dreams and challenges, the Nine Tools will open the way and enhance your understanding. They are particularly effective for learning to be a creative and relaxed parent.

Tool Time for Parenting

Just introducing imagination work into your family life bumps up the creativity quotient in your parenting style. The simple act of working the Tools with your child will relax both of you. And as you practice together, you'll naturally deepen your trust in each other.

But sometimes you might want more specific, and personal, direction—a way to gain gentle control in a challenging moment or to refine your general parenting skills. This is another place imagery can help. Perhaps you're having trouble curbing your own anger. Or old hurts are undermining your best intentions. Maybe you're frazzled and need another perspective. Your imagination is ready with more resources than you realize. One mom used the skills she acquired from the Nine Tools to diffuse her reactions to her disruptive eight-year-old. Instead of losing her temper and insisting he "act his age," she imagined him as only three. The increased patience she gained enabled her to calmly explain what she wanted from him, and her son responded well to slower and shorter directions. Another mother had an imagined conversation with her father, who had died a few years back. He told her that he loved her, something he never said when he was alive. As she shared the message, she realized how important those words were. She resolved to tell her kids daily that she loved them.

There are so many ways to adapt the Nine Tools to your parenting concerns. You've probably got a running list in the back of your mind already. Here are a few quick tips to get you started:

Listen to Your Heart and Gut Feelings: Your love and intuition are as important as your intellect in raising children. Taking time to get quiet and listen to your Heart and Belly will create a balance between what you think and what you feel, reflecting your truest self.

Talk to Your Wise Self: Grab some paper and have a "chat" with the wisest mom or dad inside you. Letters are great for this, or write with your nondominant hand. Ask what you need to know, and see what insightful answers appear.

Ask the Experts: Who is the best mom or dad you ever knew or heard of? Why not imagine her or him as your Personal Wizard? Let that individual "train" you and turn the love you have for your child into the best magic there is.

Call on Animal Allies: You can use Animal Friends just like your child does. The animal kingdom is filled with examples of great nurturing. Go to your Special Place and ask for a guide. See who shows up.

As you mix and match the Tools for yourself, you'll discover unlimited sources of strength, calm, and wisdom right in your own heart, mind, and imagination. Remember Janice, the mom with the squabbling siblings? She found new perspective after her imagery took her to a forest glen, where she saw a wide-eyed fawn and a big brown bear. "Oh no," she thought. "That bear is going to pounce on the deer!" Instead, the bear just smiled and quietly ambled away. "The Gift was that every living creature, no matter how unique, can be equal and friends," she said. That image gave her patience for her very different children and their boisterous way of settling disagreements.

I led Bonnie and her disruptive son into twin meditations in which they imagined switching places. Mom remembered what it was like to be a kid, and Paul pictured how he would feel if his own child misbehaved. They came away more attuned to each other and more in touch with their own Hearts. As Bonnie relinquished her frustration and reconnected with her love for Paul, she realized they could find their way through any problem. "I feel totally different," she told him afterward. "My anger is gone, and only my love remains. We can work this out."

And Ray tended to his grieving Heart with a simple visualization. He had a "conversation" with his dying brother, one he couldn't have had any other way. It gave him a chance to say good-bye and brought a sense of closure. After that, he was able to create more peace at home.

Peace is one of the primary goals of imagination work. Peace of mind, peace of heart, and peace at home. One of the best ways to foster this harmony is to learn my top ten list, "What Kids Most Want and Need from Their Parents."

Playing the Top Ten

Nine-year-old Allegra asked me to speak to her parents on her behalf. She had a list of concerns she was afraid to bring up, behaviors that made her anxious and unable to concentrate on her schoolwork and chores. Her requests included:

- Not yelling at each other; it woke her up at night
- Not screaming at her older brother

- Never hitting her, for any reason
- Not saying anything mean or hurtful to her
- Making it safe for her to talk about her feelings
- Being more positive

Kids like Allegra have taught me a lot about good parenting. They are much wiser than we give them credit for and know exactly what they need to thrive. Over the years, these requests have evolved into the top ten list below. I share them with adults whenever I can. Not only do these items promote stronger family ties, but they are principles that create a safe emotional context in which to teach your child the Nine Tools. If you think about the qualities you appreciated or would have liked in your parents, you may find many on this list.

What Kids Most Want and Need from Their Parents

Dr. Charlotte's Top Ten List

- ♥ Patience
- ♥ Understanding
- ♥ Listening
- ♥ Soft voices
- ♥ Structure
- ♥ Consistency
- ♥ Love
- ♥ Freedom connected to responsibility
- ♥ Family and extended family
- ♥ Role models

Patience: Things take time. It's a simple and frustrating fact of life. You want your child to learn faster, change quicker, get unstuck sooner, and move ahead in life. But kids learn and change as fast as they are able, and no faster. If you can accept that, allow yours to be exactly where she is, and help her move, slowly and steadily, toward her goals, she might surprise you. *Impatience*, and its side-kicks *Anger* and *Frustration*, actually slow change, eating up energy and time. Imagination work is a process, not a miracle. It requires patience on everyone's part. However, Tools like the Balloon Breath and a Special Place can help you keep your cool and gain perspective. After all, patience is a lifelong lesson. You, too, must start where you are and do the best you can.

Understanding: Childhood is a profound and challenging time, yet we quickly forget what it's like to be a kid. With your under-standing, your child will feel supported enough try new behaviors. Without it, he can feel cut off and alone. Let your imagination take you back to when you were ten, or eight, or five. What were you like? What crazy things did you hide from your parents? What were you proud of that they didn't understand? How did they handle it? What would you have preferred? You don't have to agree with your child's point of view. You can still impose consequences on poor behavior. But if you can at least understand how he feels and why he does what he does, you can become the true coach on his life team.

Listening: Sometimes kids need to talk. A lot. They don't want a quick fix or even a full solution. Often, unless they ask for help, they just want to know that you hear them. Even when they do ask, it's still better to listen first and solve gently. After all, how can you understand what your child is experiencing until you really hear what she thinks and feels? This quality is particularly important in imagination work. If she's to learn to trust her own wisdom, you'll both have to do some old-fashioned listening.

Soft Voices: No one likes to be yelled at, and children tell me they hear their parents' words more clearly when they use soft voices.

Otherwise, they hear the roar but miss the message. Tools like the Balloon Breath and Listening to Your Heart and Belly can center you before you speak, keeping you focused on the lesson you hope to impart.

Structure: Since much of life is unpredictable, clear boundaries, rules, and routines are comforting; they provide a dependable framework for your child's life and help him feel safe. Try to incorporate imagination time into the structure of your day or week with the same stability as bedtime rituals and family meals. Your child will come to look forward to and rely on it.

Consistency: Consistent rules, expectations, and most important, consistent behavior on your part build your child's sense of safety. She needs to trust that black won't become white between today and tomorrow. You are the anchor in her world; if you say one thing and do another, she'll lose her mooring. This doesn't mean you should be rigid; there is something to be said for flexibility in responding to new situations. But before a child can trust herself, she needs to feel secure in the world around her; your consistency will foster that trust.

Love: It goes without saying that you love your child. But it shouldn't. It actually needs to be said a lot, and also shown in tangible ways. After all, love is more than a feeling; it's an action. That sweet, sometimes painful, swell in your heart is just the starting point. How does your child know you love him? How does he experience it? Children are always translating messages from the world around them, but sometimes they're mistaken. They may misread anger or impatience as lack of love. Don't assume your child knows you love him. Keep this important gift front and center in all your interactions.

Freedom Connected to Responsibility: Freedom is an important, but complex quality. Your child needs a certain amount of it—which grows as she grows—in order to develop independence. But it must be tempered by responsibility so she can build social grace and self-esteem. It's a parental two-step: you let her go out to play with her friends (freedom) as long as she's home in time for dinner (responsibility). Learning freedom within rules creates a more harmonious home and fosters an independent child who is accountable for her actions.

Family and Extended Family: Try as you might, you cannot answer all your child's needs for love and attention. It's the impossible myth of the nuclear family. Community is a critical component of child rearing, a vital source of support for parents and children. And the core of your community is family—immediate and extended—as well as good friends who feel like family. Their love and assistance create a safety net for all of you. Maybe you can't help with history projects, but Grandpa can. When things between you are temporarily strained, perhaps your child can find a sounding board in an aunt, uncle, or family friend. There's nothing like another perspective to calm everyone down. Make the time to connect with your community. Everyone benefits when you do.

Role Models: Children learn from what you do, not what you say. You are their first and most important role model. So be the person you would like your kids to grow into. Show them you can laugh at yourself. Make mistakes, apologize, and learn from them. Reveal and honor your feelings. And consider how you can use the Nine Tools to address your own challenges and dreams. Being a good role model will teach them more than anything you ever tell them.

Put into practice, these ten elements result in healthier, happier children and a thriving family. Keep them in mind as you introduce the Nine Tools, but tailor them to your family, too. Is something important missing? Add it to the list. Maybe your child has his own suggestions. Let them open a conversation between you. Consider which of the Top Ten feel easy to you. Give yourself gold stars for success. Do any feel challenging? Perhaps you can use the Nine Tools to strengthen that quality in yourself. And don't forget this important question: How much patience, understanding, love, and structure do you offer yourself? You need these gifts, too.

The Cave of Great Wisdom
Imagery for Parent Support

Here's a guided imagery created to nurture and empower *you*. Read this aloud and record this journey for yourself, have a friend or partner read it to you, or use my CD version. But even reading it alone will produce a shift. Make sure you allow for long pauses as you go along.

We're going to take some time for you . . . special time that you deserve. As you focus on your breathing, allow your body to relax . . . Slowly, go inside yourself. Notice a beautiful, protective gold light around you, bringing you peace and calm. You are safe and ready to take your journey . . . down a wondrous road to an enchanting cave . . . deep, deep inside.

You find yourself walking along a peaceful path. There are mountains in the distance, thick with trees, and birds flying overhead. The sky is a palette of pastels. The air is fresh and bright. A stream trickles nearby.

One mountain seems to draw you toward it. At the base, there is an opening that leads to a cave. A wise Guide waits at the entrance. Perhaps it's someone you know. Maybe it's someone you have not yet met or who is no longer with you. This loving being has your best interests at heart and is there to take you inside.

As you enter together, glowing candles light the way. You are safe and protected, with much wisdom around you. Drawings and paintings cover the walls—fantastic stories and messages just for you. They illustrate your journey . . . how far you've come . . . where you're going.

Continue walking into the cave, into yourself, for as long as you need. You, too, are wise; you know what's right for you. When you are ready, allow yourself to arrive at the center of the Cave of Great Wisdom.

Before you is a gorgeous throne, encrusted in jewels. It has velvet cushions and reflects sunshine, even deep in this mountain. Your Guide motions for you to sit. As you let your body sink into the lush fabric, a procession begins . . . of family and friends whom you have touched deeply. They walk by slowly, thanking you for all you've done for them, revealing how you've helped them, how their life has been enriched by knowing you. One by one, they stop and place a Gift before you . . . a word, a thought, or something tangible. Let yourself receive them; you deserve them all. Perhaps you have not realized, until now, how much your family and friends love you, how important you are to them. Allow your Heart to respond to this outpouring.

You deserve so much . . . love, appreciation, kindness, and more. As your Heart remains open, you'll continue to receive. There's plenty of time to take it all in. You may notice that your head and shoulders feel lighter, your burdens released. As you discover and remember how blessed you are, how grateful you feel, your Heart expands.

A Wise One appears to answer your questions and reveal your next step as a Parent, the next step in your Personal Life, the next step in your Growth. Listen with an open Heart . . . all you need and want to know will be shared. Notice what Pearls of Wisdom are offered to help you meet your challenges. Ask this Wise One about anything else you'd like to understand.

Stay here for as long as you need. This Cave of Great Wisdom is always available to you.

When you are ready, come back slowly through the Cave with your Guide. When you arrive outside, return to your path. Take the time you need. Bring all the Gifts and information with you. Trust that you will remember all of it and that your wisdom will grow each day.

Become aware of your breathing, your body, your feet connected to the earth, and open your eyes slowly, feeling refreshed. If you like, write or draw the messages you received.

Taking It to the Next Step

By now, you should have a basic understanding of the Nine Tools and how to use them. Perhaps you've introduced a few to your child and are discovering their charm and power. You may have experimented with adding music, drawing, or writing into the mix. Can you feel how full your Imagination Tool Box has become?

The next part will show you how to work with the Nine Tools on specific childhood issues. Each chapter features tales of children who have used their imagination to improve their lives, as well as suggestions on adapting these skills for your family. It's a chance to see how the Tools work in real life and how, like hammers and nails, the same concepts adapt easily to different dilemmas.

As you read these accounts, however, remember that I saw these children over a period of time, and success seems easier and faster in the retelling. Some of these kids saw me for many months and struggled through the same learning curve your child may experience. Their stories are simply a blueprint for addressing similar concerns. Your child's personality and imagination, and yours, will shape your application of the Tools, as will the particulars of your situation. As I've said before, there's always a bit of improv in imagination work—but that's what makes it so magical.

PART TWO

PUTTING THE TOOLS TO WORK

Everyone Deserves to Be Happy

> The only way to love yourself
> is to believe and believe in
> yourself.
>
> —*Luke, age eleven*

How Your Child Can Be His Own Best Friend

Best friend. There may be no two words that mean so much to your child. After family, friends are among the key forces that shape her world. Watch her face when she says "my best friend." It glows.

But one best friend is more important than the rest, and that's the one inside. Not an imaginary friend, but the face your child sees in the mirror. This friendship, if nurtured, will let him weather the storms of life. Once he can be his own best friend, with all the self-love that implies, he'll be closer to solving other issues he encounters.

Self-love is like a hothouse flower; it needs the right conditions to flourish and is too easily and unconsciously nipped in the bud. All children need support and may benefit from nourishing—or reviving—a real sense of self. Children like four-year-old Sam, who thought he was unlovable because his dad left daily, even though his father was only going to work. Or Lauren, who at seven, blamed herself for her parents' arguments. They loved each other, but she thought she was horrible to make them so angry. Even kids who start out feeling good about themselves can shed those positive emotions as they grow.[1]

It doesn't take much to undermine a developing sense of self. Like thirsty plants, young minds suck up every bit of information around them, but not always with accurate results, like Sam's interpreting work absences as a lack of love. Additionally, parents, teachers, friends, and the media influence children's opinions of who they should be just as they are determining that themselves. Any disparity can damage their confidence. And then there are the normal losses, disappointments, failures, and illnesses that can blast holes in a growing self-image.

Whether the cause is a direct attack or slow erosion, without self-love, children have trouble trusting and helping themselves or connecting with others. They are more vulnerable to peer pressure, which can seduce them into poor choices like cheating and stealing, or later, experimenting with drugs, alcohol, and sex. With a strong foundation of love and self-acceptance, kids learn to value their own company and integrity over just "fitting in." They realize that they can nurture and depend on themselves. It's an astonishing and powerful discovery.

So what is self-love? It is not a tendency to think only about oneself. That's narcissism—another mask for insecurity. And it's not entitlement—the assumption that we deserve anything and everything we want. Real self-love is more complex, and it includes a deep sense of self-esteem. The California Task Force on Self-Esteem and Personal and Social Responsibility, created to coalesce contemporary research on the subject, defines self-esteem as "appreciating my own worth and importance, as well as the worth and importance of others, having the character to be accountable for myself, and to act responsibly toward others."[2] You feel good about yourself *because* you know the value of responsibility, hard work, character, and the common good. But it's a balancing act. Children need to appreciate their own worth first, or they may focus on filling a bottomless void of neediness and be unable to think of others.

Research has shown what every parent knows—each child has a

unique inborn personality and temperament. The way we respond to our children and the environment we create for them shapes how they feel about themselves. Your child needs many positive messages to develop his potential. No matter the past, you can begin building a reservoir of optimistic feelings today, starting where your kids are and leading them where you'd like them to go. The crucial qualities your child needs to become his own best friend include:

- Self-acceptance (approving of who you are, exactly as you are—body, mind, personality, and feelings)
- Self-appreciation (placing high value on those attributes)
- Positive outlook and positive self-talk
- Responsibility to self and others

Your goal is to help your child find these traits in himself, but you may need to plant and tend them first. This is where imagery steps in. The Nine Tools create a bridge between your child's imagination and his day-to-day thoughts and actions, developing and strengthening inner resources. Your child becomes the author of his own healing. The ability to find the answers inside, instead of looking to outside counsel, is an important first step to learning self-care, self-sufficiency, and self-esteem.

I Hate Myself!

How to Develop Self-Acceptance and Self-Appreciation

Six-year-old Chloe ran from the playground and hid in the bushes. She hated herself for having no friends. A dark cloud of peer rejection obscured her feelings of self-worth, normally apparent in her bubbling personality at home. Chloe felt excluded. Other girls had easily formed a close group in soccer practice, while Chloe's forte was swimming. Rejected, she didn't know what to do.

Chloe's parents reassured her that her classmates would be lucky to be her friend, but she didn't believe them. At six, she already had a history of losses. Her nursery school chum turned away from her in kindergarten. She found another friend around the block, but within six months that girl wouldn't play with her either. Each betrayal shook Chloe's tender heart. So whenever a new friend appeared, it was natural for her to worry that she, too, might leave. Chloe's fragile sense of self was in tatters. By the time her parents brought her to me, they were disturbed by their daughter's prolonged sadness.

Chloe's dilemma is common. Children begin to discover themselves through the eyes of others—first parents, then teachers and friends. And while this is natural, it's also risky. After all, peers have power; that's why peer pressure is such an issue. And small friends are fickle; everyone is learning what friendship means, and few are skilled yet. This makes the twin goals of self-acceptance and self-appreciation as vital as food to a young heart. When these are nurtured in a child, she's able to honor and express her true feelings, value her skill and creativity, balance risk with realistic expectations, and offer forgiveness. Imagery is a great way to strengthen these core components of self-love. That's what I hoped would happen with Chloe.

Chloe needed a sanctuary. Fortunately, she had a lush inner world and, when I asked her, easily imagined a peaceful refuge. She was at a beach, over which rose a magnificent orange sun with a pink heart at its center. The sky was layered in yellows, pinks, and blues; birds chipped in the distance; soft aqua waves lapped at the shore. Chloe relaxed there for the rest of our first session.

Once Rested, Time for Inner Work: Chloe couldn't rely on her friends to change; she needed something to shift in her. The next time we met, I suggested she close her eyes and focus on the Balloon Breath. Once comfortable breathing deeply, she returned to her Special Beach Place. I asked her if she noticed any animals that could help. A pink and black Crab and a spotted purple Starfish rested on the yellow polka-dotted sand. Did they have anything they wanted to show, tell, or give her that could make her feel better? Chloe imagined a Gift of a *Peach Music Box* with a dancing figure on top. Anytime she had upsetting or angry thoughts about herself, they would disappear into the box.

QUICK TIP!   **No Fixed Order for Using Tools**

Although I often start kids off with the Balloon Breath, Chloe skipped it and went directly to finding a Special Place. Only then did I show her how to calm herself with deep breathing. Sometimes I might teach two or three Tools before returning to the first. Be flexible.

Water Washes Worries: As Chloe explored her Special Place over several visits, she discovered if you "dip your hands in the water, your troubles go away." This Special Place soon became her favorite daydream. She always found a present there with notes like, "I love you" and "You're special," and new Animal Friends to meet. Once, a kind Deer delivered an important message from her parents: "We love you."

Hearts Offer Understanding: One week, Chloe was feeling particularly blue because her classmates had ignored her at lunch. I suggested she check with her Heart. She drew it, misshapen and outlined in black, with charcoal scribbles covering most of the pink areas. A smaller heart, broken, black, and chipped, was inside the larger one, with a sad little kitty crying inside. This heart was shut tight. When I asked her, Chloe admitted that the last time she had allowed love into her heart was in preschool.

Black Heart Transformed: Chloe was desperate for love from her peers, but she needed to learn to love herself first. What to do? I had her ask her Heart for advice. First question: What color is *Love*? "Pink!"—her favorite color. I suggested she breathe pink Love into her Heart, filling it up as much as possible, and notice what happened. In a few minutes, Chloe reported that it was now smiling and open, surrounded by gold. One half held the little kitty, brought to vibrant life with popping ears and tail. The other side held two more hearts, one with an open door to let Love in.

Treasure Worth Digging: With her Heart in much better shape, I asked Chloe about its message for her. She returned to her Special Place and sat under The Tree of Trust. As I led her into this reverie, I suggested that if she found a shovel beside the tree, it could help her dig up a treasure box that held an answer. With the assistance of a friendly Panther, she started digging and found a black jewel-covered box with a key attached. Inside were great riches and a letter from her Heart. The note said she had a good life with friends and family. There were just a few false friends she didn't need. Its final message— "Love Yourself."

QUICK TIP!   Underground Treasure

There are things your child just doesn't know, even about himself. Digging for treasure is one way to see what's below his awareness. How hidden or difficult the treasure is to reach can be an indication of how far beneath his awareness his answers lie. Chloe's treasure was deep but not miles down, and she was able to access wisdom she wouldn't normally encounter on her own. Your child can do the same.

Escapades with Owls and Wizards: Over the next few weeks, Chloe had many more adventures. She met a wise Owl who helped transform her disappointment into the confidence she needed to reach out to girls at school. Then she bumped into Sparkle, a young Wizard who lived in the Hut of Hugs. Sparkle came equipped with three crystal Gifts: A heart-shaped crystal helped Chloe love herself even after her friends snubbed her; it also kept her Heart strong and kind around the girls who rejected her. A star-shaped crystal made her feel like a star, no matter what. Here, Chloe was learning to validate herself without depending on unreliable peers. Finally, as if she were preparing for future challenges, Chloe received a diamond-shaped crystal that "could help with everything."

Backtrack Alert

Sometimes young imaginations need a push. You might have to be directive in your instructions until your child catches on or if he becomes resistant to helping himself. For example, he might find a Gift but not understand its significance. That's when you can suggest asking an Animal Friend the meaning of the Gift. Or maybe invisible ink is involved, requiring special light for him to see what's written. No matter what block your child encounters, you can offer something to help him through. Once he's mastered his Imagery Toolbox, it'll be easier to say, "Go inside, ask for help, and see who shows up." He'll take it from there.

Open Heart Works: At one point Chloe wondered if she had imagined that her friends were excluding her. When she returned to school the following Monday, they seemed perfectly happy to have her join them. Chloe had tapped into a profound life lesson: What we tell ourselves—good or bad—affects how we see the world and, in turn, how the world sees us. Or as this bright six-year-old wisely put it, "Your heart can be open or closed. If it's closed, it's probably mad and not in a good mood. And if it's open, you're happy to get love."

With that, Chloe forged confidently ahead. She had connected to her inner wisdom and found Tools to heal herself. She made new friends, and when they wanted to play with others from time to time, she no longer took it personally. One of Chloe's last drawings was a big chart entitled "I Love ME!!" She listed the qualities she was proudest of—helpfulness, creativity, and humor. It was a literal *sign* of self-appreciation and self-worth. She also included her personal reminders for happy Heart.

> **EASY HINTS!**
>
> **How to keep my heart open . . .**
>
> **CHLOE'S CLUES**
> 1 Go to my Special Place when I feel lonely.
> 2 Wash away sad thoughts.
> 3 Remember Mommy and Daddy love me.
> 4 Listen to my Animal Friends; they know a lot.
> 5 Think Pink! It makes my Heart smile.
> 6 Expect people to be nice.
> 7 Don't worry about mean kids.
> 8 Say, "I love you, Chloe" every day.

HOW-TO FOR YOU

Chloe is a fine example of how a child builds self-love. Here are some ideas for yours:

Create a Safe Sanctuary

Have your child imagine a Special Place where he can feel good about himself. He can surround himself with whatever and whoever gives him respite from his troubles. This breather can provide new perspective and the possibility of a better self-image.

❖ Consult with an Animal Friend

Once he has found his Special Place, ask your child to notice any wise animal guides who are there to help him learn to love himself. You might ask:

- What does your Animal Friend look like?
- What message does your Animal Friend have for you?
- What Gift does he give you to feel better about yourself?

❖ Imagine New Scenarios

Enlist your child's imagination to envision different realities. For instance, if he thinks he doesn't have friends, have him create a scene where he does. Ask how *that* feels. Who is around him? Are there kids from his class he might have overlooked? If he has difficulty, use your own imagination to help him create a setting where he feels supported and loved.

❖ Connect with Heart Wisdom

Help your child connect to his Heart's true feelings, even if they are uncomfortable. Have him imagine what his Heart looks like, feels like, and wants to say about loving himself. This will help him start to trust his own emotions, which is an important step toward trusting and appreciating himself.

❖ Add a Touch of Whimsy

You can create fun labels like Chloe's Tree of Trust and Hut of Hugs. It lightens the learning. Younger kids might enjoy Rooms of Love or the Spaceship of Specialness; older ones may prefer Private Point or Quiet Quarters.

❖ Consider Wizard Wisdom

Suggest your child call in Wizard Wisdom if he needs super-self-love support. Wizards pack a powerful punch when other imagery Tools fall short.

⠿ Plant Seeds of Self-Appreciation

No soil is as fertile as a child's mind and Heart; your every action sinks in and quickly takes root. Show your acceptance and confidence with phrases such as: "I like the way you did that." "I know you'll do fine." "This is hard, but you'll get through it."

My Life Is So Awful!

How to Cultivate a Positive Outlook and Positive Self-Talk

At eight, Deidre seemed to have everything—she was brilliant in school, a natural artist, an amazing dancer, and she sang like a lark. But something inside was off. Deidre's attitude had soured—on herself, her loving parents, and her life. It seemed to have happened overnight, but it had been building for months.

Deidre had a long list of complaints: "My body looks weird. I hate my life. I have too much to do. I'm jealous of my little brother. My friends don't want to play with me. I don't feel like eating. I hardly see my dad. I can't sleep. I have nothing to look forward to." She wrote notes to her parents about ruining their lives because she was such a terrible daughter. They didn't know what triggered such negative thoughts and were quite disturbed.

What we say to ourselves matters, even when no one hears it but us. Words have the power to create and destroy, to inspire and depress, and the ones we tell ourselves shape our lives as surely as hands on soft clay. Consider the fascinating work of Masuro Emoto, who studied the impact of speech and thought on water crystals and rice. In an experiment with school kids, he put cooked rice in two jars and had the children speak to them. They said angry, hurtful things to one jar and kind, loving words to the other. The negative jar turned brown and rotted; the loving jar did not.[3] If harsh words can suck the life out of rice, imagine what they do to our spirits.

Imagery, however, can reverse this trend. Wise Animal Friends and Wizards who show up to help are, after all, creatures of your child's own making. They are born in a deep part of the imagination that maintains hope, no matter what painful outer events transpire. The Gifts and messages of a child's own wisdom are more potent than any outside counsel and were what Deidre needed to restore joy to her life.

Locked by Tension: When I first met Deidre, she admitted she felt pressure to be perfect. This stress seemed to turn her against herself. I wondered what the pressure felt and looked like, so I suggested that she go inside and see what picture formed. Deidre envisioned herself with locks on her shoulders, hips, and feet. Could anything release such suffering? We invited in a loving animal guide. A Monkey sat next to a shady tree, holding the key to Deidre's locks. Nearby was a pile of locks he'd already opened.

Feelings Run Amok: Once that initial pressure released, Deidre began to experience and express negative feelings she'd been hiding for some time, like anger and aggravation. She had held them in whenever adults said anything that upset her, but now they overflowed. Over the next couple of weeks, she hit her babysitter, was nasty to her mom, threw tantrums, and awakened crabby. Although it seemed as if Deidre went from good to bad to worse, this was neither unexpected nor unusual.

Backtrack Alert

External calm isn't always real, and when negative feelings are buried, they can harm the child who hides them. Bad feelings need to emerge. Getting in touch with your child's hurt and anger is healing; it's the first step in his taking responsibility for his true feelings and expressing them in ways that don't hurt himself or others. This takes time and is not always direct. Hang in there if he, like Deidre, needs to release bottled-up emotions. With your patience and guidance, he will eventually find his calm.

Loving Corrections Misconstrued: Deidre's parents had asked her to be a bit more positive and to alter her hurtful behavior. But she couldn't handle anything that felt like criticism. Even if her parents spoke calmly, she heard them screaming. Her need to be perfect convinced her that if she did one thing wrong, everything was wrong, and she was a terrible person. This anger at herself extended to her parents. And despite the unlocked pressure, Deidre suffered from a painfully closed and unforgiving heart.

Releasing the Unforgiving Heart: When Deidre looked inside again, she discovered the middle of her chest was filled with intertwined red and brown wires. Her vulnerable Heart was wired shut. She claimed she couldn't forgive her parents for criticizing her, but I sensed that it was her reaction to her parents' corrections that were causing her distress. Deidre really had to forgive herself . . . for her negativity, her poor behavior, and most of all, for her normal imperfections. Only then could she move on. When I asked if she could forgive herself, she was open to the idea but didn't know how. I suggested she imagine which colors represented *Self-Forgiveness.* She breathed pink and purple into her Heart, and the tangled wires began to separate; slowly, her *Anger*, *Sadness*, and *Jealousy* left.

Deidre checked back in with her Heart. It was now a healthy, multicolored pink and red. "It's as if all my bad thoughts went to the bottom of my heart and got smaller and smaller till they disappeared," said Deidre, "and all the good things floated to the top." This realization helped her start to feel more positive about herself.

Loving Energy Shifts Patterns: Two weeks later, Deidre was distraught again. She was unsure if she should be negative or positive about her life; she straddled the old thoughts and the new thoughts, with nowhere to land. Her drawing illustrated the problem perfectly: on one side of the page, she drew an angel, and on the other, a devil. A big black X separated them. Blotches of black paint all over the paper showed her distress. We did a combination of imagery and energy work that day. Soft music played in the background as she calmed herself with her Balloon Breath. I centered myself as well. Then I placed my hands in her energy field, three to six inches above her body. I imagined myself pulling out her bad feelings and replacing them with love.

We didn't speak, but afterward she told me, "When your hands were over my heart, I heard it talking. 'Don't be negative,' it said. 'Think of happy things.' When your hands moved over my belly, a voice whispered, 'Things will be okay. Don't worry.'" When I reached her legs, Deidre felt the bad feelings being sucked out. And when I got to the soles of her feet, she felt dark spots on her left foot, but also light entering, exploding the blackness. And she felt an angel nearby, ready to comfort her in whatever challenges she faced.

Like a blocked well, Deidre's dark feelings had prevented her good feelings from reaching the surface. Once she felt the energy release her negativity, she could experience the goodness that was there all along. The encouraging voice and angel she imagined seemed to remind her that healing and forgiveness were possible.

Deidre then painted four brightly colored hearts: a large one for each parent and smaller ones for herself and her brother. The title: "I LOVE MY FAMILY." When I saw that, I knew she had discovered an important truth: that hearts can be broken by bitter words, but they can be repaired and reconnected to the love underneath.

Bring in Positive Self-Talk: I wanted to support Deidre as she became more open and positive about her life. I suggested she talk to herself. Not out loud, but inside. I asked her to replace the sad/bad/mad thoughts with happier ones. We brainstormed and came up with five easy sentences she could choose from:

1 I am peaceful and loving.
2 I get along easily with my family.
3 I solve problems fairly and smoothly.
4 I love and appreciate myself.
5 Life can be fun.

Deidre asked how often she needed to say nice things to herself. I directed her back inside to find the answer that worked best for her. The formula popped right up—three times a day, three times each.

Writing Works Wonders: In another imagery session, Monkey reappeared and gave Deidre a Gift of a *Shiny Pen*. Deidre found relief in writing long letters to her mom. It was a brilliant way to let Mom support her. After school, late at night, anytime big emotions overcame her, Deidre charted her feelings—sad, confused, silly, even happy—and her life continued to improve.

. . . So Does Drawing: Monkey's advice also helped Deidre address her negative emotions. "If you're feeling sad, drawing makes it better," Monkey told her. "If you are angry, you can let it out, too."

The shiny pen made her pictures come alive, and that small miracle helped her feel better. One day Monkey showed up with a blue, green, and pink pencil that had a magical eraser. "It erases my bad thoughts about me," Deidre explained.

Final Transformation: After months of work, Deidre created an inner garden with edible flowers of beauty and love. As she imagined slowly chewing them, I suggested that the flowers could fill her Heart with love, then extend that love throughout her body. The deep peace it brought reinforced a positive outlook. The flowers also sent messages when she was down on herself: "Don't think nobody loves you. Don't think you're ugly. You're beautiful and terrific." And a sturdy Turtle reminded her that she had everything she needed to know—to love and be nice—right inside. She only had to check with her Heart and ask. Deidre had learned to build herself up from the inside out. Her final words to me were, "I prefer to be happy. I hope other kids do, too."

HOW-TO FOR YOU

Deidre used imagery Tools to restore her positive view of the world. Here's how you can help your child do the same:

⠸ Practice Forgiveness

Encourage your child to forgive himself as well as others. Have him imagine what forgiveness looks, feels, or sounds like. Is it a color, a feeling, a character, music? Have him bring whatever he imagines into his Heart and notice what happens. He can ask, "What do I need to do or understand before I can forgive. . . . my parents, my friend, myself?"

Very young children may not understand the word "forgiveness," but they understand "I'm sorry." Explain that sometimes people do things that make you sad or mad, like when a friend breaks a toy or steps on your toe. When they're really sorry, and you can accept their apology and be friends again—you are forgiving them. Use examples from his own life, moments where he offered or received forgiveness, and he'll catch on soon enough.

Harness Paper Power

Suggest he put his negative view of life—his dark feelings and thoughts—on paper. Drawing and writing can be cathartic, a release of your child's angst. Or perhaps he would like to dance or sing his feelings. Once he can let go of his negativity, it will be easier to create a positive outlook. Next have him draw how he'd like his life to be, and see what emerges.

Use Gifts Wisely

Allow your child to enjoy and use whatever Gifts he receives. Some kids have been given special glasses to see the bright side, precious stones to remind them how special they are, and magic mirrors that show them their real beauty. Trust that any Gift your child imagines will be a positive pointer on the path of self-love.

Play with Color

Have him experiment with the wonder of color. See how breathing different colors in and out alters his gloomy feelings—from anger to calm, from frustration to love, from a closed heart to an open one.

Share Loving Energy

Your love for your child is powerful medicine. Share it with him by sending love from your Heart to his. Or visualize love traveling from your heart, down into your hands, and into your hugs. See if he can feel it. Practice together.

❊ Talk to Yourself Inside—Nicely

Sometimes we have to practice talking positively about ourselves and others. Have your child think of one or two nice things to say about himself, family members, and friends. Make an ongoing list and stick it on your fridge as a reminder.

❊ Praise Progress, Not Perfection

Kids can mistakenly connect "getting it right" with getting love and may berate themselves for anything less than perfection. Help your child recognize small victories and how far he's come. By focusing on his efforts and improvements, success becomes a rainbow of possibilities.

It's Not My Job!

Responsibility as a Two-Way Street

Luke was an eleven-year-old with a big problem. He felt responsible when anything went wrong and thought it was his job to make everyone happy. When his younger sister stole cookies, he took the fall. When his older brother threw a baseball and shattered a window, Luke said he did it and accepted a two-day restriction as punishment. When a school buddy cheated on a test, and his teacher asked Luke what happened, he confessed: "It's my fault Bill cheated; I let him see my work." Luke thought he shouldn't be forgiven for anything and often called himself an "idiot." He wrote to his dad: "I'm sorry for all the problems I cause you."

Responsibility is one of the hallmarks of self-love; it includes accountability for our decisions and actions, attention to physical and emotional health, cooperation with others, and acting with a sense of values and integrity. These qualities are among the building blocks of self-worth. They are also challenging. Responsibility is like learning to ride a bike; you can fall before you're steady. Imagery Tools are wonderful training wheels. They give children creative ways to address the feelings and obstacles that slow their progress and to accept that taking responsibility is not always easy.

Luke might seem an unlikely candidate for this section since he had an overdeveloped sense of responsibility toward others. However, self-love begins with the Self. And by focusing all his energy on others, Luke ignored himself. We want our kids to think of others, but not to their own detriment. This means they must face their dark places before their kind acts represent true caring. Luke offers us an example of how one boy used imagery to take care of himself, then extended that self-love outward.

Don't Ignore Yourself: When I met Luke, he felt so poorly about himself, he ignored his own needs. He thought by taking responsibility for others, he was doing the right thing. The irony, of course, was that this behavior was neither good for Luke nor the people he was "helping," since his actions interfered with lessons they had to learn about telling the truth and making good choices. In this case, self-responsibility, taking care of himself, trumped social responsibility, taking care of others—at least until he could do both honestly.

QUICK TIP! Caring For Yourself First Is Okay

It's the old airplane advice: Put the oxygen mask on yourself before you help your neighbor. There is nothing wrong with being kind to others—it's a very important trait—so long as your child doesn't sacrifice her own emotional or physical well-being in the process.

And Don't Hurt Yourself: What struck me most was Luke's tendency to turn on himself. Instead of a strong inner base, which would let him bounce back from mistakes, the smallest infraction sent him into a tailspin. Some kids brush off misdeeds as nothing. They are able to apologize and go on. Not Luke. He blamed himself for everything.

Remember a Favorite Vacation: In light of Luke's guilt, I thought an important first step would be to create a safe place. First we relaxed his body with a waterfall of white light. Then he chose a vacation spot in Mexico with jungle-like pools and lush waterfalls. When he became lost with so many pools, his beloved dog, Oscar, joined him. Oscar, who had recently died, became Luke's guide, showing him the way out of the imaginary "jungle."

Backtrack Alert

Sometimes, when a child looks for a safe place, the unexpected shows up, like when Luke got lost in his Mexican oasis. That's okay. It just indicates where your child is right now. To help her move through these obstacles, simply use other imagery Tools, like an Animal Friend, to face the dilemma at hand.

Take a Trip to Inner Wisdom: I suggested that Luke imagine following Oscar beyond the pools, along a path, until he reached the Forest of Inner Wisdom. There he met a "really old" Wizard dressed in a silver cape and red tunic who immediately touched Luke's Heart with his magic wand. This touch gave Luke the Gift of *Kindness*, so he could be nice to himself. I recommended that the Wizard lead Luke into a cave that housed the Wisdom Library. He introduced him to the librarian, whom Luke imagined as a 500-year-old Elf. Her extreme age suggested lots of life experience and good judgment.

Books Are Resourceful: Elf found the perfect book for Luke. It had a cracked leather cover with gold-edged pages and was called *How to Love Yourself.* Luke opened the book and read, "The only way to love yourself is to believe and believe in yourself." The book spelled out how: "Think about your goal and believe it every day, every night, every second." This was wonderful advice. By focusing on his goal—to treat himself well—he was more likely to learn ways to take care of himself before attending to others.

Reliable Snake Wisdom: His Wizard's wand then transformed into an emerald green snake with piercing black eyes. Most kids would jump at the sight, but Luke was fascinated. Snake gave him a silver charm that contained a picture of a contented, calm Luke. Snake's job was to remind Luke to wear his pendant and never give up. He was on his way.

Time Flies When You're Trying to Take Care of Yourself: A setback came when Luke claimed he didn't have enough time—not even to think about doing something nice for himself. I suggested he ask for help. As soon as he did, another Snake appeared. Across his fangs, he carried a gold watch on a chain; it would give Luke the time he needed to do kind things for himself daily.

Backtrack Alert

Your child might create excuses for not taking responsibility for himself. Resistance is common. Keep addressing each problem with an imagination solution, and she'll get through it.

Love Me . . . Love Me Not: I still wondered if there might be a part of Luke that didn't want to take good care of himself, so I asked him to see if that was true. Yes indeed. Cloud of Brown Smoke lived in his right leg and was a masquerade for *Fear*—a belief that all this work was for nothing. We needed a powerful force to rescue him.

Brain Belief Factory Follows: I encouraged Luke to go back inside and ask for assistance. A Super Belief Wizard showed up. Dressed in the same red tunic as Luke's original Wizard, but with neon green hair, he came bearing Super Belief potion. To determine how much was needed, he took Luke deep inside Luke's own brain to The Belief Factory, where all his notions were created. They found that only 20 percent of his "belief in himself" was working. To pump up that percentage, Luke felt that the ideal dosage was one drop a night for each bone in his body—206 drops in all (a recently learned science fact). This medicine increased Luke's belief in himself from a "4" to a "10" out of 10!

Listen to Your Elders: Luke also connected with the adult Luke, the one who had learned to love himself and take responsibility for his actions years ago. He was successful with a happy family, and more flexible than the child Luke. From twenty years in the future, he had come back to offer support. His message? "Erase your bad thoughts and never give up."

Soon, Luke was taking more and more responsibility for his feelings and actions—both in being kind to himself and to others. And with much more honesty. He stopped sabotaging his own success just to help someone else. He was stepping into his power.

HOW-TO FOR YOU

Your child can use imagination strategies to step into her own power and responsibility.

Find Happiness and Let It Grow

Invite your child to imagine what brings her joy. Brainstorm together. Make sure there are lots of no-cost happy activities like spending time at the park with you, playing with dolls, or going to the beach. By bringing simple delights into her daily life, she'll start learning to be responsible for finding her own happiness.

Put on Your Oxygen Mask First

Encourage your child to use polite words and do caring deeds for others, as long as she is also good to herself. Make a success list and add one new item daily. A few achievements might include:

- Brushed my teeth without being reminded.
- Checked in with Heart and Belly twice today.
- Did homework before watching TV.
- Helped Mom do dishes.
- Shared my dessert with Suzy at lunch.

Discover Wisdom Within

Take your child to the Forest of Inner Wisdom. Have her ask whomever she meets there—magical beings, forest creatures, even the plants themselves—"What do I need to know to be kind and loving to myself? To my family? My friends?" Have her keep an eye open for Gifts. Remember, she has wise answers inside; she just needs a nudge in the right direction. And you know the way: through the Balloon Breath, down her path, just a little bit right of somewhere.

Face the Shadow

Light and dark, up and down, happy and sad . . . so much of life comes in equal and opposite pairings. But when it comes to feelings, we tend to view down and dark as failings, instead of what they really are: the other side of the emotional coin. It's important for your child to explore her dark side and accept thoughts and qualities that aren't so terrific. We all have them, but we don't have to act on them; acknowledging them is plenty. It's easier to say, "Hi, revenge. I know you're there, but I'm choosing to stay calm," than to pretend it doesn't exist.

▪ Connect with Your Wise Elder

Have your child imagine herself as an older, wiser self, with lots of life experience. What would "she" advise? You might be surprised at how much she sounds like you.

Loving Yourself from Day One
Imagery for Becoming Your Own Best Friend

In the following guided imagery, your child imagines himself receiving all the love he wants and needs, in just the way he wishes. This creates an opportunity to repair some of the natural bruises of childhood, no matter his age or the source of his hurt. Parents aren't perfect . . . or omniscient. As much as we love our children, we may not express ourselves in the exact ways they want to be loved. This exercise lets your child begin to rewrite history. It's all the more powerful because it comes with your understanding and consent. Envisioning what it feels like to have already received every bit of love and understanding he could possibly desire will strengthen his inner core of love, worthiness, and appreciation for himself, and will increase the likelihood of his becoming his own best friend.

Gently close your eyes and breathe slowly. Get comfortable. We're going to take an imagination trip. First, picture a beautiful day on a pleasant path. Imagine that you can turn around and walk back in time.

Let's go back to last week. Or last month. Remember something fun that happened. Keep walking back . . . all the way back to last year, or the year before, maybe during the holidays or your birthday. Recall something special about those days.

Take yourself back even further, back to preschool, to playing with your favorite toys, enjoying Mom at home, or running in the park with Dad. Let something that feels good stand out from that time.

Now let's go all the way back to the day you were born. Imagine being welcomed into this life. Ask yourself if there is anything you would like to change. How do you want to be loved and accepted as you grow up? Go ahead and change it. Create exactly what you desire.

Imagine being cherished from your first moment on earth. Notice how thrilled and blessed your parents feel to have you in their lives. See yourself as truly tiny, held perfectly and gently in their arms. They shower you with love and attention, more than your heart could desire, so you are completely filled. You deserve it, just by being you and coming into this world. Allow yourself to have all the love that you ever hoped for. Really feel and see it, so you can take these thoughts and feelings with you.

Picture yourself growing from day one to year one. Imagine your mommy or daddy holding and loving and caring for you just the way you want. And all your parents' words are spoken with kindness, gentleness, and warmth.

Imagine love continuing to pour in as you grow. You are accepted and loved, and you grow healthy and strong. Your heart is filled with peace and joy and confidence. It's in your heart to be kind to others, to help others, to get along. These wonderful qualities are part of you now . . . as you go to preschool . . . to kindergarten . . . as you grow up.

So grow yourself up. Imagine yourself just six months ago, and see how well you're turning out, having received love the way you want. And bring yourself to the age you are now. Notice any differences, since you have received exactly what you needed and wanted while growing up.

Take yourself into your future and see next week, or next month, or next year . . . doing well, being happy, having fun, getting along with everyone, helping your family and friends, facing any problems you meet with confidence. Now take a giant leap into the way far future and imagine yourself all grown. Imagine having a wonderful life, whatever you choose to do. You feel so comfortable with yourself, and you have the skills to work for what you want, for your heart's passion. Take time to enjoy what you've created.

Now you can give yourself the love you want and need, with each breath and each thought. You can always return to the beginning, reimagine your life, and receive what you need. You have that power. When you're ready, bring yourself back into present time and slowly open your eyes.

When Life Is Making Your Kid Sick

Reducing Stomachaches, Headaches, and Other Aches

> Instead of having stomachaches and headaches, I learned how to feel my feelings. My feelings are okay.
>
> —Jones, age eight

★ Do you ever get stomachaches or headaches?" Each time I walk into a classroom and ask that question, almost every child raises a hand. Then all the kids start talking at once, telling me about their aches and pains and how much they'd like relief. Five-year-old Jasmine's nervous tummyaches caused her to miss a lot of school. A swarm of black, purple, and red butterflies were trapped inside her, fluttering madly. No wonder she was nauseous and sore. Shane's father's recent surgery had upset his own health. Throughout his dad's long hospital stay, the ten-year-old had kept his feelings inside, telling his parents that he was fine. But his body told the truth in the form of throbbing headaches.

The emotional challenges of life often take a toll on growing bodies. Almost half the kids I see have stress-related physical issues, and studies show that 30 to 40 percent of children report pain at least once a week.[1] Their headaches, stomachaches, and tics appear when the last straw lands on their small camel backs. Kids can take just so much life pressure before something "breaks." Stress is the culprit behind many of the frequent headaches, stomachaches, and other physical symptoms that plague children.[2]

Anxiety, fear, and worry can also affect the immune system—indeed all cells of the body—often resulting in distress and disease. For instance, most children experience stomachaches at some time. But chronic stomachaches (known as Recurrent Abdominal Pain, or RAP) affect 10 to 25 percent of all school-aged children. These kids tend to miss lots of school, playdates, and family functions. Only 5 to 10 percent of these stomachaches have a physical reason.[3]

When we're under pressure, the primary stress hormone, *cortisol*, slows down important processes, including digestion. It delays aspects of our immune response, increasing vulnerability to infection. Cortisol also creates inflammation by releasing another chemical, *cytokine*. That's good when we have a puncture wound because inflammation is critical in tissue repair. But when there's nothing to repair, stress creates chronic inflammation. This can exacerbate skin conditions and trigger asthma attacks.

Imagery, however, can diminish stress and the physical ailments it causes. Positive images have a tremendous impact on pain when children are in a relaxed state.[4] Focusing on personal imageries can distract them from discomfort and allow their bodies to rebalance. It also gives kids a way to explore and express the hidden feelings that cause stress. They can learn to control pain levels, reduce physical tics, and eliminate warts. And they can use relaxation and imagery to help with the discomfort of asthma, nausea, and medical procedures.[5]

In one university study, 85 percent of the children showed improvement in symptoms after six weeks of using imagery CDs at home; 35 percent were pain-free, compared to 7 percent in the control group.[6] I see those same transformations in my office. In one imagery group, three kids came in with three different ailments: a headache, a stomachache, and a painful canker sore. To ease their suffering, we went to a magical garden where they could plant anything they wanted, including seeds of health. While their inner garden (their body) was growing plants and flowers, they lounged in a healing pond where their pain could dissolve. When the journey was over, the headache was gone, the tummy felt fine, and the canker sore didn't sting. In fact, the boy with the sore practiced the healing pond imagery all week at home and reported that it went away in three or four days instead of the usual seven.

Medication is not always the best treatment for childhood aches, especially when stress is a factor. The Nine Tools can relieve many of your child's common complaints, while also teaching him to manage his own healing.

Of course, sometimes nothing helps but a warm water bottle on a tender tummy or an ice pack for an aching head. While imagery Tools can be used on immediate pain, they also work well between bouts of distress, as part of a prevention program. The benefits are cumulative, and once your child learns to use her imagination and intuition, they will become trusted members of your emergency first aid kit.

Now let's take a look at how to help your child reduce pain and heal some common ailments, including:

- Stomachaches
- Headaches
- Tics
- Warts

You can easily transfer the skills learned here to other health situations.

When Stress Affects Your Belly

How to Cope with Cramps, Stomachaches, and Other Unwanted Tummy Symptoms

Alisha was an intense third-grader. She couldn't tolerate loud noises or changes in routine. She was also a high achiever, pushing herself at school and in sports. But while other kids let problems roll off their backs, Alisha became disturbed and anxious. When she felt overwhelmed, she had trouble sleeping and couldn't problem-solve clearly. And if she didn't give or get 110 percent, she called herself a "loser."

Her sensitivity made her vulnerable to cramps, diarrhea, and constipation. Alisha's parents had already taken her to a nutritionist, who eliminated milk and wheat from her diet. Homeopathic medicine, vitamins, and acupressure were also tried. A pediatric gastro-enterologist suggested antidepressants. Except that Alisha's parents wanted to help her help herself.

It's always important to have a doctor rule out serious, underlying issues. But relaxation and imagery can promote better digestion and reduce cramping whether they arise from a true physical cause or upsetting emotions.[7] That's what we were counting on with Alisha.

When I first met Alisha, she told me straight away, "Everything would be perfect if I didn't have this stomach stuff." She lamented her symptoms and worried about bathroom availability whenever she was away from home.

High Stress a No-Go: As we talked, I wondered if her school and social concerns were causing tension in her belly. Alisha agreed that her high stress level might be hurting her, so I had her focus on slow deep breathing. I asked her to turn inside to see where her stress resided. Using her imagination, Alisha scanned her entire body and found a large, square, black block of cement in the middle of her brain. It was such a startling discovery that I had her draw it.

Make It More Real: In the drawing, the outline of Alisha's body was off-center and out of balance. The stress box took up almost her entire head. I advised her to search for an antidote; she found

Calmness in her shoulders, expressed as lavender swirls. She breathed these calm feelings into her hands, neck, and head. Her stress began to melt and travel down to her toes, where it dissolved out her feet. Then lavender *Calm* shifted into pink *Love*, filling her body. When Alisha redrew her self-portrait, her body was now solid and grounded.

Avert Tummy Attack: We then focused on specific situations that might set off a stomachache. Alisha was worried about an upcoming softball tournament. I asked her to check in with the wisdom of her Heart and Belly. What would help her address her worry? They told her to use the body scan technique she had learned earlier.

Repeat Body Scan: When Alisha scanned again, she found *Nervousness* in her knee; it was "chicken yellow." I suggested adding *Confidence* to her repertoire of positive coping skills. Calmness now moved into her left pinky and changed to green, while Confidence became lavender and took up residence in her right thumb.

....

Backtrack Alert

....

During imagery, feelings, colors, and positions may change—just like in life. Help your child stay true to himself and be honest about how he feels in the moment, always allowing for shifts. Besides, he won't get confused—it's his inner landscape.

....

Blending Resources Adds Impact: I asked Alisha to imagine breathing the green Calmness and lavender Confidence from her hands down into her nervous knees. As she did, her apprehension began to fade: they worked together to create a new color—copper. With this stronger, metallic knee, Alisha could overcome any worry.

Five Animal Friends Arrive: One week, Alisha came in anxious about the school play. She called in some Animal Friends. Five showed up. Deer brought a punching bag to help release her frustrations; Alisha hadn't gotten the part she wanted and almost refused to participate. Bunny offered a pillow to rest her head on, since she was nervous about forgetting her few lines. Parrot brought blue calming pills and reminded her to do Balloon Breaths. Dog invited Alisha to feel at home on the stage and gave her the Gift of *Smiling*. And Cat gave her a gold necklace with three diamonds to strengthen Calm and Confidence.

Take Homework: I sent Alisha home with Good Health Homework. She was to practice her Balloon Breath and check in with her Heart and Belly every day, as often as necessary. These would help her stay calm under stress. I also reminded her to call on any of her guides—Wizards or Animal Friends—for support.

A Letter of Thanks to a Wizard: Alisha did her homework diligently, and when she needed extra help, she contacted her Wizard on her own. Soon she began feeling much better. Her thank-you note shows how far she'd come.

> *Dear Wizard,*
> *Today you did your part, and I did mine. We worked together when I was worried because I couldn't remember my lines. Then I did my Balloon Breaths, and asked you what to do. You said to get help to practice my part. That would calm me down. It helped a lot. In no time, I did great!*

Rainbow Lake Brings Relaxation: After some months, Alisha's Wizard went on vacation to Hawaii and she had to take charge of her own health. She created Rainbow Lake, where all feelings were welcome. She imagined herself floating on a raft. On either side, ribbons of color represented a wide range of emotions, from nervous yellow, sad blue, and angry red, to tickled pink, happy orange, confident green, and copper strength. Rainbow Lake became a safe place to doff her shoes and expectations—to float, relax, and allow her belly to heal.

QUICK TIP!   **When Helpers Leave Town**

> Wizards take vacations. Animals Friends tend to other business. Everyone deserves a break. If this happens with your child, it might mean that he's gaining the skills to do more for himself. However, if he still lacks confidence, have him visualize a stand-in. It might be a Wizard-in-training or an Animal Friend's cousin. Another helper is just around the corner of his imagination, ready to be called in.

At the end of our work together, Alisha felt confident enough in her healing to offer advice to other kids on overcoming a nervous belly: "If you really, really listen to what your brain and your Heart say, and you do your Balloon Breaths, the very nervous you gets to be calmer—and it helps a lot."

HOW-TO FOR YOU

Alisha's strides in taking charge of her tummy woes can spill over to your child. Here are some ideas to try.

⊞ Focus on Stress—and Apply Its Antidote

Have your child create a picture in his mind (or on paper) of his stress. What does it look like? Is it in his belly itself or somewhere else? Then let his imagination conjure what will dissolve it. *Joy? Calm?* Another strength? Help him breathe in that antidote and see what happens to the pain in his tummy.

❖ Take Another Look at Stress Situations

Discuss possible triggers for tummy distress (like an upcoming test) and what Tools he could use to prevent it. Will imagining his Special Place calm him? Should Confidence Wizard be at his side? Then play out a new scenario—this time with a positive outcome.

❖ Blend Colors for New Outcomes

Just like the colors in a paint box, feelings and energy colors can be combined for different and often stronger results. Alisha mixed green *Calm* and lavender *Confidence* to create a new color, copper, and a new feeling that was at once calm, confident, and powerful. Your child might discover that red *Happy* and purple *Brave*, combined, can more effectively combat the yellow *Worry* that grips his belly than either one alone. Encourage him to experiment.

❖ Invite a Slew of Animal Buddies

During role-play or real stomachaches, invite the assistance of Animals Friends and Wizards to help your child discover what he can do to alleviate pain. Does he need to rest more? Drink more water? Speak up for himself? Admit that he's scared or sad, so feelings don't get stuck in the belly? Your child's inner wisdom will call in the right helpers to provide soothing Gifts and sound advice. Follow their counsel.

❖ Find His Rainbow Lake

Support your child in finding his own relaxing Special Place, somewhere he can visit regularly to keep his stress below tummy pain levels.

❖ Do Good Health Homework

Have him ask his Heart how often he should go over what he has learned. Then pick a good time to review. If you plan to work with him, he's more likely to practice, especially in the beginning. His Heart may be wise, but sometimes brains forget. By practicing together, you can remember for both of you until his new tummy-tamers become a habit.

▪ Cuddle Your Child

If he feels loved and supported, his hurt won't bother him as much. Anxiety worsens pain. So hold, rock, and hug your child.

When Pressure Pains Your Brain

How to Manage the Tension Tigers of Headaches and Migraines

When Ethan's parents walked through my door, they had come straight from their pediatrician. Their ten-year-old was having awful headaches, including migraines that caused dizziness, nausea, and vomiting. Ethan feared he might have a brain tumor, although CAT scan results were normal. In a bad month, he could miss a week of school. He was taking medicine for these frequent head-pounders, but it wasn't always effective. Nor did the doctor want him to rely on medication. She felt Ethan needed to learn to relax and overcome his stress. His parents believed that Ethan's headaches were caused by either emotional issues or undetected physical problems that would require sensitive support. Either way, this led them to me.

Headaches are the most common pain kids have. Ninety percent of all school-aged children experience them,[8] and they are often associated with high levels of pressure and anxiety. They may be caused by specific events, but could also be the result of underdeveloped coping skills. Life is stressful and not everyone can roll with the punches.

Tension headaches result when stressed-out muscles in the head or neck start squeezing too hard. Kids describe this pain as steady and dull or like a tight band around their heads. Migraines afflict 10 percent of all children. They usually affect one side of the head, although children can experience them on both sides or across the forehead. New research shows that migraine sufferers have unusually excitable nerve cells. When a migraine is triggered, these cells suddenly fire electrical impulses that ripple from the back of the brain across the top, then back down to the brain stem, where critical pain centers are located. The "wave" of electrical impulses causes blood flow to increase drastically then quickly drop off. The inflamed blood vessels can create intense pain that kids describe as pulsating or throbbing. It can last for hours or days. Migraines run in families, so if you have them, your child has a 50 percent chance of getting them, too.[9]

Migraines are more likely to be set off by the following:

- Eating patterns and sensitivity to foods such as chocolate, caffeine, cheese, and sugar
- Too little or too much sleep
- Light and sound sensitivity
- Stress
- Emotions, especially feelings of anger or perfectionism
- Lack of exercise or overexertion
- Changes in barometric pressure

The good news is that headaches can be helped, and often without medication. Naturally, you always want your doctor to rule out serious physical problems. But whether the source is physical or emotional, imagery can be a cool answer for hot heads, doing double-duty in your creative medicine cabinet. The Nine Tools can help your child unravel the tangled nerves and tight muscles that result in chronic headaches and, at the same time, learn tension-taming skills that last a lifetime. Soothing today's bad headache may help prevent or lessen tomorrow's. That was certainly the goal with Ethan.

Ethan's headaches had begun at age seven, and his pain caused him great worry—as if he were spinning out of control. The headaches could last twenty-four hours. Occasionally, he awoke with one. Ethan's mom suffered from migraines, and his grandfather had tension headaches, so there was a clear family history. That made Headache 101 a good place to start.

A Little Education Can't Hurt: Ethan and I talked about what he believed caused his headaches and, in particular, his migraines. I educated him about common migraine triggers. This became an opportunity for him to better understand what may go on in his body when headaches arrive and how he might prevent them.

Headaches Defy Description: Ethan described some of his headaches as pounding cannonballs; others felt like "humungous pliers" gripping his temples. He created a character for his headaches: a muscular hard-hat construction worker wearing a T-shirt, announcing he's a "Bad Guy." He held an enormous drill in each hand and opened the top of Ethan's head, drilling directly into the brain. The intense pain made Ethan weep. "I wish I was dead."

SWAT Team: Extra-strength Tylenol sometimes helped, so I asked Ethan how he imagined the drug worked. He drew a picture of Tylenol as a little paratrooper leading a SWAT team that flew into his brain to rescue him. I suggested he ask the little guy to help him often, even without the medicine. Ethan practiced this image repeatedly. And over time, he found it soothed him.

Journaling Brings Awareness: I also encouraged Ethan to keep a headache journal. Whenever he experienced pain, he was to note the date, time, and level, along with what he was feeling before the headache started, both from that day and the day before. Ethan discovered that his *Anger* was "like fire exploding," and *Worry* was a "dark blue mouse" frantically scurrying in his head. The visual connections between his headaches and anger, stress, and frustration motivated him to practice the Balloon Breath.

Headache Head-On: One day, Ethan came into my office with a pounding headache. Until that moment, I had not seen him in the throes of one, but now he was suffering. His eyes were sunken, and the energy had been drained from him. I chose the Three-Question Exercise for quick relief. This simple visualization and relaxation technique helps a child monitor and report the changing color, shape, and weight of pain. It's a simple process, but it short-circuits all kinds of physical discomfort.

QUICK TIP! Three-Question Exercise

This imagery may relieve or eliminate pain. Start with the Balloon Breath (preferably with eyes closed). Have your child note exactly where her pain is. Then ask . . .

1 What color is it?
2 What shape is it?
3 How heavy is it?

Any answer is okay. Be accepting and positive, using words like "good," "fine," and "okay" after each response. Have her continue the Balloon Breaths three or four times between questions. Let her simply visualize and report. Continue to ask these three questions in rounds. The answers will likely change as she relaxes, and the pain often becomes lighter and smaller. How many rounds you do will depend on your child's openness to relaxation and the intensity of her pain.

Healing Process: We worked the Three-Question Exercise for ten to fifteen minutes, and Ethan's headache changed from dark (black then red), sharp (square then triangle), and heavy (10 tons) to pale (light blue to yellow to white), round, and insubstantial (1 pound). Although Ethan was in a lot of pain at first (8 on a 10-point scale), by the end of this exercise, his headache was at a mostly manageable 3.

QUICK TIP!

0 to 10 Scale

This scale is commonly used to judge pain levels in medical settings, but it's a great tool for children in all kinds of situations. It allows them to rank any feeling or experience from 0 (nothing) to 10 (the most they can imagine). Once they establish the level of their experience, they can apply imagery and then recheck to track progress.

Ask the Source: I asked Ethan to have a conversation with his headache to find out what he needed to know, do, or understand to release any remaining bits of pain. His headache told him that he was stressed and needed to slow down. He then told me about his day—rushing through lunch without enough to eat or drink, then a fierce basketball game—and we realized that all this had made him dehydrated and thrown him off balance.

Melt Away the Rest: With this awareness and an agreement to take better care of himself, Ethan imagined his pain melting through his temple and out of his head. I held my hand about three inches from his forehead to give him a direction in which to send his pain—out and away.

Explore the Depths: About a month later, Ethan reported that he had had another terrible headache. Because he wasn't in immediate pain, we revisited this experience as a discovery mission. Ethan imagined his headache as a deep black lake. When I asked if he could go into those waters to learn more, he dove right in. The waters got warmer as he swam into the core of his headache. Inside was a gold star. Before Ethan understood the meaning of the star, the water got unexpectedly hot. He needed to swim to the top of the pond for safety, and just before the red and swirling torrent reached the boiling point, he escaped.

Call In a Health Wizard: When I asked Ethan about the meaning of these intense images, he said, "The star is my headache, and it's sending out hot vibes through my head." But he couldn't explain the dangerous, boiling waters or what to do about them. It was time for extraordinary guidance, so I suggested Ethan ask for Wizard Wisdom. Almost immediately, a Health Wizard (HW) appeared. He wore a sleeveless blue diving suit, camouflaging him in the water. But he had been standing by all along. Ethan asked him the meaning of the hot waters. HW explained that the temperature increased as Ethan's headache got stronger.

Ethan asked for help, and HW assured him that he'd send a signal before a headache came on. It would be a small voice in his head or a feeling in his body reminding him to slow down, breathe, and imagine holding a cool ice rock to his head to prevent pain. And HW promised that if Ethan found himself in that hot lake again, he would have a waterfall appear to cool him.

That year, Ethan's headaches and migraine symptoms decreased considerably.

EASY HINTS!

How to relieve awful headaches . . .

ETHAN'S EPIPHANIES

1 Keep a headache journal and tell the truth.
2 Remember to drink lots of water.
3 Don't skip meals.
4 Practice the Balloon Breath every day to relax.
5 Use different colors to cool down a boiling head.
6 Check in with my Health Wizard and take his medicine, even if it seems weird.

He didn't need as much medication and managed to attend school regularly. He even made a list of healthy habits for other headache sufferers (page 119).

HOW-TO FOR YOU

Ethan overcame so much in learning to better control his headache pain. Your child can, too.

Learn About Headaches

Teach your child about the common causes of headaches and ways to prevent them. She might not know how important it is to drink water in hot weather or how stress tightens muscles in her head, neck, and shoulders.

Describe the Headaches

Have your child create an imagination picture for her headache. Depending on her age, she can draw it, you can draw it, or she can simply describe it verbally. What does it look like? Feel like? Be specific. What she envisions will be a clue to understanding how to gain mastery over her pain.

Use the Power of the Other Hand

Writing can offer wonderful insights, and engaging the nondominant hand often elicits surprising results. Assign your child's nondominant hand to speak for her headache, while the dominant hand asks questions. After she chooses one color to represent her pain, and another one to soothe, help her begin the interview. She might start with, "Hello, Headache. I'd like you to stop hurting me," and then have the other hand respond. Let them "converse" for a bit to see what information is revealed. Finally, have her ask the key question: "What do I need to know or do to stop the pain?" Remember, this is a tool for older children who are comfortable writing. Younger kids will gain insight more easily from speaking with a Wizard or wise Animal Friend.

⠵ Pay Attention to Feelings

Encourage your child to be aware of her feelings throughout the day. This will help her learn the difference between headaches caused by physical issues such as hunger and those caused by emotions (anger or frustration). Periodically, check in with the 0 to 10 Scale to see where she is and how much she can lower her stress level with imagery.

⠵ Keep a Headache Book

Let your child keep track of her healing journey by putting together a simple headache journal. She can write down when a headache occurs, how long it lasts, pain level, what emotions preceded it, and what Tools she used to help herself. Younger kids can draw and dictate what they want to say. Writing and drawing out her feelings and thoughts will show her which emotions and life situations contribute to her stress, and which Tools offer the most relief.

⠵ Add Energy Healing

Put your hand three to six inches from the source of pain. Imagine pulling out the hurt and releasing it through the back of your hand. If any pain remains, encourage your child to send it through your palm as well.

When Life Creates Other Symptoms

How to Handle Unwanted Tics and Warts

At six, Ben was an active gymnast. His body loved to move, and he was an Olympic hopeful. But two years earlier Ben had developed a variety of tics—chest tapping, nose twitching, eye blinking, throat clearing, hair twirling—although not all at once. Sometimes coughing and clearing his throat were predominant; other times, he rubbed his nose. Not only that, poor Ben had warts. Ben's parents had chalked up the tics to his vibrant activity level, until his first grade teacher questioned them. And the warts? They were just bad luck.

More and more parents come into my office concerned about their child's nervous habits. Kids do their best to hold it all together, but overwhelming stress often speaks through their bodies as repetitive physical habits. These brief and involuntary motions or sounds, like flipping hair, flapping hands, blinking, coughing, or whistling, are as unconscious as they are persistent. They are also common. Five to twenty percent of all schoolchildren will have tics, and boys are four times as likely to experience them as girls. Most children outgrow them. But if a child has severe problems that last more than a year, combine motor and vocal tics, and impair social or academic functioning, she should be evaluated for Tourette's, which affects about three percent of children.[10] Imagery, however, and its cousin, hypnosis (which uses more directed suggestions), have been shown to decrease the incidence and severity of tics.[11]

Stress can also increase vulnerability to another unwelcome childhood issue—warts. Up to 50 percent of all children develop warts. They are caused by a common virus (*human papillomavirus*, HPV). By depressing the immune system, stress chemicals may make kids more vulnerable to HPV. Imagery can actually help warts disappear. In one study, a seven-year-old girl used imagery to eliminate eight of sixteen facial warts within two weeks, and eighty-two more on her face and body within three months.[12]

When I met Ben, we decided to address the body movements first; perhaps they were related to strong feelings he didn't know how to express. We began by tracing his body on large sheets of paper and we went on a visual pilgrimage to discover where he kept different feelings. Ben closed his eyes and noticed where they seemed to be. What emotion was in his eyes? Where did he put frustration?

Life-Size Drawing Reveals Much: He chose a variety of glittery crayons, smelly markers, and 3-D glue paints. Together, we colored the feelings he encountered—mad, sad, glad, weird, and wired—on his body outline. I then wondered if he would like to let go of some that he no longer needed (like *Worry* in his eyes). Perhaps he could accomplish this simply by breathing it out? And maybe he could add more of the feelings he did want—like *Happy* and *Glad*—by breathing those in? Ben was willing, so we gave it a try. That released some of his stress. It was a good start.

QUICK TIP!　　　**Turn a Half-Blind Eye**

It's tempting to address your child's nervous habits when they show up, usually by asking her to stop whatever she's doing. Unfortunately, this direct approach often backfires by increasing the symptoms. These are, after all, stress-related behaviors, and undue attention adds stress. When I see a child tapping her foot or chewing her nails, I simply suggest we do Balloon Breaths. That tends to calm her for a while; then we can address the nervous habit in a safe and healing moment.

Warts Add Worry: Ben had several warts on his face and hands. He didn't like people staring at or making fun of him, but as we talked, it became apparent that he also viewed his tics and warts as awkward friends. They were familiar. He didn't know who he would be if he wasn't constantly moving his body or rubbing his warts. He wasn't willing to let them go, but he did agree to relax a bit. He was terrified of the dermatologist's dry ice treatment, so his imagination was open to other options.

Animal Friend to the Rescue: I suggested Ben call in a trusted companion. Parrot flew into town and gave Ben the Gift of *Yellow Medicine Dots.* They were "like little bombs that hit and killed the warts." When applied to his face and hands, the warts dissolved into nothing. Instructions were to use them twice a day for two minutes each. A supply of orange dots was extra powerful but had to be used sparingly. Both helped some.

Not to Worry When Warts Return: Ben made progress with his warts; in a few weeks, several disappeared. But then some returned. So Ben went inside and asked the warts what to do. He learned that he needed to breathe in *Calmness* (green and blue) and imagine the warts going away again. He was to do this twice a day for fifteen days. Ben practiced this exercise for three minutes when he woke up, and before he went to sleep. And telling his warts to "Go away!" empowered him.

Freeze Away with Ice Cream: To boost effectiveness, I led Ben through an ice cream freezing imagery, a different technique than he would find in his doctor's office. We audiotaped an exercise for him to practice at home each day after he centered himself with the Balloon Breath. Here's the sample script.

SAMPLE SCRIPT — **Freezing Warts with Ice Cream**

"Imagine your favorite ice cream or other frozen dessert in a cup. Remember its color, flavor, smell, and taste. Picture that with every slow deep breath, the cup gets bigger and bigger, filling up with more yummy ice cream. Now think about putting some of this ice cream on the warts. Wow is that cold! You can really feel your warts freezing. As you continue to Balloon Breathe slowly, the freezing cream shuts off the blood supply to your warts so they can't live anymore. The warts dry up and fall off. Take your time. (*Wait a minute or two.*) You can hardly feel anything in that spot now. There is as much ice cream as you need for your skin to be clear and smooth. Just start your slow Balloon Breath, remember your favorite flavor, and wherever you have any warts, put some on."

....

Help at Healing Pond: We then stopped at a healing pond to give Ben a chance to rest and rejuvenate. He imagined cool green healing waters that he could float in or drink to heal himself inside and out. Every cell in his body was cleansed and healthy: there was no room for viruses. And Ben was so relaxed he didn't need his tics.

Treasures Await: Ben's healing pond was also filled with Gifts and treasures. I asked if any of the Gifts could bring him *hope* that his body could feel better. He noticed bright goldfish right away. Swimming across his chest, arms, and hands, they surrounded him with the Gift of *Hope*. Then I inquired what could help him *believe* this could happen. Ben swam deep down to the bottom of the pool, where shiny green stones gave him the Gift of *Belief*. And when I wondered what might help him feel *strong* enough or *brave* enough to help his body, he found purple powder sprinkled on the edges of the pond; it gave him *Strength* and *Courage*. With these Gifts, Ben felt wise and capable of handling anything.

Setbacks to Be Expected: Ben really improved over the next few months. He stopped blinking, and many of his warts disappeared. Then an innocent fishing trip retriggered an old, familiar tic. While Ben was on the boat with his dad, several fish were killed before his eyes. His shock and horror translated into constant blinking. His shame over being part of the poor fish's suffering was almost too much for him to bear. I had Ben imagine what he'd say to the fish if they were with us. Eyes closed, he told them he was sorry. The fish replied it was okay because Ben ate them, and they became part of him. This helped him come to terms with the event, and his blinking subsided.

By the time Ben left counseling, he had made great strides. The blinking, sniffling, and throat clearing had diminished, as had his warts. He learned to take time to center himself with three to five minutes of gentle Balloon Breathing three times a day. And he was learning to express feelings in words rather than body movements.

HOW-TO FOR YOU

Once your child learns these techniques for tics and warts, she'll help herself with minimal assistance from you.

Do a Body Scan

Pull out that poster paper for your younger one and trace her entire body. An older child can draw her body outline in any size she chooses. Have her identify and sketch where her tics and warts show up, giving each symptom a face or character. Do the same for stressful emotions that can exacerbate this problem. Where in her body does each feeling live? What does it look like? Draw those as well. It's a great way to begin getting in touch with what's going on inside.

Talk to Tics and Warts

Have your child tell her symptoms what she wants: "Go away now!" is a good start. Then listen to what they reply. Find a way to work together.

Talk to Stressful Feelings

Stress and uncomfortable emotions also have something to say for themselves. Unexpressed, they may act out as tics and warts, but once they start talking, they often know just what they need to feel better and go away.

⚏ Invite in a Favorite Animal

Have your child call in an Animal Friend or two and see what advice or Gifts they bring to help relieve her symptoms. They may bring magic medicines to heal the tics or dissolve the warts. They might also bring Gifts to address the feelings behind the problem, like an antidote for anger or a talisman against worry or stress.

⚏ Try the Ice Cream Cure

Use the sample script on page 124–25 to help your child "freeze" away warts. If she doesn't happen to like ice cream, any cold treat will do. Ice cubes or a pile of snowballs are also popular. It's much more fun than a trip to the doctor, and often as effective.

Creating Your Inner Garden and Healing Pond
Imagery for a Happy, Healthy Body

The following meditation is beneficial for any kind of physical ailment. The lush, growing garden represents the physical body and your child's ability to cultivate health. The healing pond is an inner sanctuary where your child can receive all the healing that the mind and imagination can offer. Children don't need to understand this metaphor to reap the benefits of the journey. Like a fairy tale, it works best on a subtle, subconscious level.

Allow your eyes to gently close and focus on your breathing as each part of your body relaxes and your troubles begin to float away. Imagine walking on a path of loving light with gorgeous flowers around you, sweet smells, and birds singing in the distance. In front of you is a big, beautiful gate that leads you to your own healthy and magical garden. You look under a nearby rock and find a key with your initials carved in it. You know this is your gate and your key.

A wise Wizard appears from around the gate to help you grow your inner garden. What does your Wizard look like? What kind of clothing is he wearing? How does your Wizard smell? How does your Wizard smile? What does your Wizard say? Notice everything.

Go in the gate and begin to create your garden. You have everything you need—all the tools and seeds, lots of little plants and flowers, and some young trees, all ready to be placed in the ground. And you have all the food and water to nourish and nurture yourself and this beautiful place. You may even plant seeds of health, joy, peace, and calmness, or any other qualities you would like to have so that your body can be totally happy and healthy. Your Wizard will help you with this.

In one part of this garden, there is a wonderful healing pond. Notice where it is, and go over to it. As you step into the water, which is the perfect temperature, you see a sleek long rock with soft, fluffy moss on it. You can use this rock as a pillow, so you can relax in the pond and keep your head out of the water. Or you can dive in. As you rest in the healing waters, they wash over you and soothe your body and your feelings. Any hurt or tightness melts away—in your heart, in your mind, in your body, in your spirit. All pain washes away.

Your Wizard has prepared some magic healing tea that reaches and cleanses the deepest, darkest places inside you. You are healed inside and outside, and you are brought back to health. What a wonderful place to be as your garden grows!

Once you are ready, step out of the healing pond and dry off. Your garden has turned into the most magnificent place. When you take the time to plant seeds in the garden, and to care for them, just like you take time to love and care for the health of your body, miraculous things can happen.

Your Wizard points out one precious flower that is calling to you. Lean down and smell its fragrance. Notice what color it is, how big it is, and its special shape. The flower whispers an important message to help you be as healthy as possible. It's time to remember to love and accept yourself totally and completely. Remember your ability to heal yourself with your positive thoughts and relaxation.

Continue to rest here for as long as you need. You may come to this garden, this healing pond, whenever you want extra relief.

CHAPTER 7

The Bogeyman and Other Scary Stuff

Overcoming Fears and Feeling Safe

> **When my wizard waves his feather around, it makes all my fears disappear and all the bad better. That's because his feather is all about love, and hope, and kindness.**
>
> —*Rose, age nine*

★ Most kids get scared. Going to the doctor, separating from Mom in kindergarten, taking exams, and watching a scary movie are typical triggers. While it's normal for a five-year-old to worry about leaving her mother, when a preteen still has trouble, there's cause for concern. Other fears arise from traumatic events—a death in the family, a hurricane, or sensationalized news reports about war and violence—can launch deep understandable anxieties. However, when they last for more than a few months, we must pay attention.

Some fears are healthy and guard us from danger. A child who is afraid of being hit by a car is more likely to look before crossing the street. But fear can also exaggerate the potential for danger, heightening worry about things that may never happen. After one ten-year-old saw a TV report about a home robbery, he refused to be alone in any room and was scared "bad people" would break in despite the protection of four barking dogs and an alarm system.

Sensitive children may perceive different energies around them and may develop seemingly unreasonable fears, such as the bogey-man, vampires, or "the monster in the closet." All are archetypal fig-ures from what philosophers and psychologists call the "collective unconscious."[1] Such receptive children can also adopt their parents' fears. One mom, who was terrified of flying, wanted her daughter to feel comfortable in an airplane, but the girl absorbed her worries and ended up in my office to overcome this terror.

When we are threatened, the *amygdala*, the emotional part of our brain that responds to fear, triggers chemical signals (adrena-line) that makes us alert to danger and ready for action—the "fight or flight" response. In caveman times, this behavior was adaptive—it protected us from death. Today there are far fewer such emergen-cies, but our minds can react as strongly to harmless situations as life-threatening ones. In these circumstances, the rational part of our brain, the *prefrontal cortex*, may shut down, leaving the amygdala to prevail.

Unaddressed fears can paralyze a child, preventing her from activities she loves. They can also trigger destructive behavior and cripple emotional growth. Your challenge as parents is not to elimi-nate fear, but to help your child become strong enough to face its powerful forces. You don't have to know where a fear comes from—sometimes you can't—but it's important to validate your child's feel-ings, and teach him skills to manage them.

His imagination offers effective solutions for moving through and beyond fear. Consider five-year-old Liam, who decided to cork his fears in a bottle. He threw the bottle in a can, clamped a lid on it, then tossed the container into another dimension to make it vanish forever. And after meditating, eleven-year-old Rebecca bravely stood up and sagely noted fear is the emotion "absolutely everybody" has to deal with at some point in their lives.

In this chapter we'll be addressing five common developmental fears: abandonment, the unknown, doctors, disasters, and dying. Let's look at several children's experiences, how they overcame their fears, and how you can help your child do the same.

What If Mom Won't Come?

Fear of Abandonment

Casey was an angelic seven-year-old from a creative family. He was athletic, articulate, and funny. Except at 2:45 every afternoon. That's when he would panic. He was terrified his mother would fail to pick him up from school. Casey saw the carpool lane from his classroom window and started worrying fifteen to thirty minutes before the bell. It didn't matter that she usually showed up on time, anticipation of even a short delay—five or ten minutes—triggered a churning stomach and trouble breathing.

Abandonment is a primal fear, the core of separation anxiety. It often has its seeds in infancy or early childhood when we are totally vulnerable and need our parents for safety and survival. When a caring adult responds to our cries, we develop feelings of security. We learn to trust the outside world, which is critical for learning to trust ourselves. But if an infant cries and no one comes quickly, he might believe that no one will ever come. And if this pattern continues, the result can be an insecure, chronically anxious child.

Separation anxiety can also develop when a good bond is established between baby and parent, as in the majority of families. It's a built-in protection to ensure children will stay close to parents, an instinctual safety mechanism—the caveman's dangerous lion is today's dangerous stranger. Children usually grow out of it as they develop better thinking and survival skills. The problem comes when they don't. And some children are naturally more anxious than others, making them more vulnerable. Ultimately, how we handle fear of abandonment is what counts, as Casey and his family came to understand.

When I first met Casey, he had no resources for understanding his fears; he was simply frantic. Inside my office, in a calm and neutral atmosphere, he learned to confront his worries through his imagination.

Create an Image: I invited Casey to close his eyes and use the Balloon Breath to center himself. Then I asked him to sense where his fears were located in his body. *Fear* and *Worry* lived in his stomach. Fear was petrifying him, Worry was terrorizing him, and both were paralyzing him. "You're never going to be picked up," Fear would say. Worry would chime in, "She's never going to remember you." During art, his favorite and last class of the day, the voices created an endless loop so he couldn't concentrate.

. . . and Draw: Casey drew Fear as a long, menacing red creature with bared teeth, one eye glaring and the other patched. Worry, attached to Fear, was a "pathetic, vomit green" figure. Creating these characters comforted Casey; when you face your fears they aren't as scary.

Have a Conversation: I had Casey converse with these wormy beasts. "Stop bothering me!" he told them. When he asked what they needed to go away, they echoed our previous conversation. "Do the Balloon Breath," they said, explaining that it would put them to sleep—but only for a day. So he decided to do his deep breathing *every* day.

Kids Repeat What You Say

Don't be surprised if your child uses your exact phrasing as she makes the Nine Tools her own. Kids frequently use the language they hear right from the start, like Casey, whose monster told him to do the Balloon Breath. Because your child is just learning these terms, they may be fresh in her memory.

Wash Away Your Fears with Color: I asked what color might lessen his fears. He said breathing in a "nice disgusting pink" would send Worry to sleep more quickly. Fear needed a slightly different formula— "pink with blue and reds, a tutti-frutti color." It worked. Casey learned that deep breathing with colors each day put his fears into deeper sleep more quickly. And they were less likely to wake up, too.

Feed Your Fears: Fear and Worry were also hungry. They had a weird and wild craving for corn, Casey's favorite vegetable. All Casey had to do was imagine giving them corn and they would calm down. But not creamed corn. Creamed corn made Fear and Worry stay in his belly for the rest of his life! He had to be careful.

Backtrack Alert

Kids can set up seemingly self-sabotaging situations. Casey's unconscious awareness that his fear and worry could stay forever reminds us that children usually don't make troubles disappear immediately. Problems can creep back in, if only for a little while. We get used to them; they become familiar. That's all part of the process. Keep working with your child until you get to the bottom of the issue, find a way to resolve it, and help her get back on track.

Say a Final Good-bye: What removed Fear and Worry once and for all? Casey realized they were just "renting space" in his stomach. When he asked, he learned that their rental agreement would last one more month. It was a sign that our time together was ending. Casey had developed the courage to ask them to leave "for good." And he knew he had to continue his deep breathing with "pink and tutti-frutti" colors—just to make sure they stayed away.

HOW-TO FOR YOU

You can follow a similar recovery roadmap to help your child conquer fear of abandonment.

Create an Imagination Picture

Encourage your child to develop a visual image for her fear of being left or forgotten. If nothing comes, ask a few simple questions:

1 In what part of your body do you feel your fear?
2 What does your fear look like (color, shape, size, weight)?
3 What other picture pops up about your fear?

Draw the Fear

Putting an image on paper makes her abandonment fears realer and yet less frightening than keeping it inside. The fear is less likely to grow when there is a concrete picture to work with.

Use Color for Healing

Suggest your child ask her fear, "What color would make you stop bothering me?" Then have her breathe that color into the fearful area. Continue the breathing for up to three minutes. Thirty seconds can seem like an eternity to a child, so be encouraging and make simple comments from time to time, such as: "Good . . . keep going . . . that's it . . . well done." Ask her to notice what happens. Often her worry about being away from you will shrink, disappear, or be covered by the soothing color.

Strike a Bargain with Fear

Have her ask, "What do I need to know or do to make this worry about Mom not being there go away?" If the response seems insurmountable, help break the instructions into more manageable steps. She can interview the feeling with the following prompts:

1 "Why are you trying to get my attention by scaring me?"
2 "What are you trying to teach me?"
3 "How can I make friends with you?"
4 "What's the first thing I need to know (or do)? The second? Third?"
5 "I don't understand what you are saying (or showing me). Make it simpler."
6 "Please slow down. The information is coming too fast."

Ask for Your Child

If your child is reluctant to dialogue with her fear of abandonment, you can ask your own intuition on her behalf. Close your eyes, focus on your Balloon Breath, and see what answer pops up in your imagination. Pass on the information you receive to see if it feels comfortable and real to her.

Parents Can Step In

Not all fears are unfounded. Some children have experienced a real sense of abandonment. Death and divorce upend a child's feeling of security. And chronic lateness can leave her wondering if she's worth remembering. Unfortunately, death and divorce may be unavoidable, but do try to arrange your schedule to be on time. If you're late, call ahead or have another trusted adult go in your place. And if trust has been broken in the past, now is the time to rebuild it. You can . . . by being there when she needs, and expects, you to be.

What Will Happen Tomorrow?

Fear of the Unknown

Eight-year-old Paulo was an intuitive and wild little guy—a mix of contradictions in a small, neat package. He was the sort of kid who would fearlessly fly through the air with the latest snowboarding technique yet tremble in the dark. His fear? The unknown. Paulo's sensitivity to change caused his stomach to crimp into wire-thin knots of pain.

Fear of the unknown can come in many guises: the dark, being alone, or change. Paulo was afraid of them all. Although the unknown can be a breeding ground for fears, it is also a fact of life. We all have to face it, and so do our kids. But children, unlike adults, lack the experience of surviving new situations, and they often feel helpless to handle them. This kind of fear is a perfect opportunity to stretch and grow, as Paulo did.

Do a Different Kind of Brain Scan: Like many children, Paulo was fascinated with the brain. So we decided to see what was happening inside his. No scary MRIs for us; this kind of imaging—through his imagination—was much more personal.

Paulo described and drew a "guy looking in to see how I feel." There was a lot going on. Buttons in various colors of red, blue, green, and yellow controlled different feelings. One little "helper man" announced: "He's mad!" In another part of his brain, a second helper noted whatever had been upsetting Paulo ". . . is back!" And still another reported some sort of explosion and circuit breaking in the lower part of his brain.

Ask for Help: The following week I asked Paulo to focus on his Balloon Breath and turn inward. After a few quiet minutes, he received a clear message: "The way to work the controls is through meditation. It makes the little brain cells feel better, and they make me feel better." That Paulo connected the Balloon Breath with meditation didn't surprise me; I knew his parents were regular meditators, and he had probably seen them do something like it. His own wise counsel, however, was much more effective than any suggestion from them or me. In fact, he went on to receive further instruction on managing his worries: "In the middle of being upset, it's good to do the Balloon Breath and focus on the love in your Heart."

QUICK TIP!   **Meditate**

Meditation does not have to be a big fancy technique used only by Eastern mystics. Balloon Breathing is a basic form of meditation. So are concentration exercises, quiet walking, running, and dancing. Almost anything that stills the mind and brings your awareness to the present moment can be a form of meditation.

Draw Your Feelings: The following session, I had Paulo explore the source of his discomfort when he faced an unknown situation— whether it was a new environment, a sudden change in schedule, or finding himself unexpectedly alone in a room. He drew a shady character, the "guy who makes fears," attacking his brain. Paulo's cartoon nemesis had a pointed head and sharp yellow teeth, with green for the whites of his eyes. "This guy chews on skin inside the body," Paulo explained. "He makes your brain send horrible, awful messages to your stomach." That's where the stomach pain comes in.

Backtrack Alert

Paulo often uses "you" or "your" instead of "me" or "my" in his descriptions. It might seem like he's detaching from his feelings. But occasionally it's easier for children to distance themselves from powerful insights. Let your child express herself in the way she's most comfortable.

Bring in the Troops: Our next step was to see if the angry creature could help. I suggested Paulo ask, "What gets rid of you?" He kept receiving the same useful advice—"meditation." Over the next few weeks Paulo also checked in with many Animal Friends: a talking Dolphin, a laughing Chimp, and a speedy Cheetah. "They tell me to center and concentrate," he explained. "They also tell me what colors to breathe in to calm myself, and what there is to learn."

As Paulo grew more confident, he shared an insight beyond his years: "Fears teach you lessons. When you're afraid, they get bigger and bigger. But if you face them, they get littler and littler. Meditating with the Balloon Breath helps get rid of the bad guys."

HOW-TO FOR YOU

Like Paulo, your child's imagination can help her face the unknown with calm.

Picture the Monster

Drawing is a great way to turn the feared unknown into something tangible and more manageable. Once your child can see his fears on paper, he can discover creative ways to let them go, including asking what they need to leave.

✲ Wisdom Outweighs Fear

Encourage your child to breathe deeply and ask his Heart and Belly for advice on handling unfamiliar or unexpected situations. For instance, "How can I feel safe? What can I do to be brave? How can we turn off my fears?" The same imagination that feeds his worries will know the perfect antidote.

✲ Animal Guides to Help

Suggest your child request an Animal Friend to assist with this fear. Ask the following questions and add your own, depending on the information and images she receives.

1 Who turns up?
2 What does your Animal Friend show or tell you?
3 What does your Animal Friend suggest you do?

Please, Not Another Needle!

Fear of Doctors

Jordan was an athletic, confident, and optimistic eleven-year-old. She handled the stress of several moves and her divorced parents' frequent disagreements like a trooper. But when it came to facing any medical procedure, she was, as she admitted, "a total wimp." And now she needed three teeth removed for braces. In her dentist's office, with local anesthetic, the procedure could be simple—except Jordan was petrified.

Medical procedures and surgery can terrify children; routine check-ups can cause panic. Fear of pain and lack of control, often rooted in early vaccines or other medical experiences, can send kids into hysterical crying, aggressive and acting-out behavior, or withdrawal to a fetal position. Imagery can return a sense of control to facing medical challenges. Jordan needed to learn how.

Practice Makes Perfect: Jordan was a softball star who knew the value of practice. Through Balloon Breathing, Jordan put herself in a self-hypnotic state and went to her favorite Special Place—the well-worn track of a local mountain footpath. This relaxation helped her feel in charge. She practiced every day, several times a day, for two weeks. But with her high anxiety, she knew that just simple deep breathing to keep calm on "needle day" would be difficult.

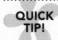

QUICK TIP!   Use Self-Hypnosis for Self-Control

Hypnosis (or self-hypnosis) here is not the strange "clucking like a duck" that we've seen in shows. It just means being extremely relaxed, aware, and open to suggestion. In self-hypnosis you give yourself specific direction, much like an affirmation: "As I approach the dentist's office, my fear disappears and I feel brave and strong." Or, "When the doctor gives me a shot, it feels like a butterfly kissing my skin." Even little kids can learn it.

Create a Body Anchor: It was critical for Jordan to access this calm on a moment's notice, so I taught her to pair touching her wrist with feeling peaceful. The connection, or anchoring, prompted her to go into a tranquil, deeply relaxed state. During our session, these suggestions went into her subconscious, increasing the likelihood of an automatic relaxation response at the de ntist, and enabling her to face whatever she must.

Gather Medical Information: I suggested Jordan's mom learn from the dentist what to expect. Understanding what would happen, from the minute she walked into the medical building gave Jordan some comfort. It helped us design an imagery experience, limited unwanted surprises, and created a feeling of being more in control.

Practice Some More: With rehearsal, Jordan gradually became more confident. First in my office, then in her home, she imagined going through all the steps of the procedure, using several senses to make her visualization as real as possible: "What does the dentist's chair feel like? How bright are the lights overhead? What is the sound of the dentist's voice as he explains what he's doing?" By facing her fears a little at a time, she slowly desensitized herself. She also listened to my Healing Pond CD each night as she practiced calming herself; it helped prepare an atmosphere for a quick recovery.

QUICK TIP! Imagine It's Already Happened

Let your child imagine how he feels after the medical procedure. How proud he is of himself. How great it all turned out. How surprisingly easy it was. Be detailed and specific in your suggestions.

EASY HINTS!

How to survive scary doctor's visits . . .

JORDAN'S PRESCRIPTION:

1 Practice my affirmations twice a day for the whole week before my appointment.
2 Imagine how GOOD I'll feel when it's over. Practice that, too.
3 Pack my relaxation CD in case I need it.
4 Use the Balloon Breath to stay calm.
5 Ask Mom to plan a treat for after!

On the day of her tooth extraction, fortified with hours of imagery practice and a CD to help her focus, Jordan willingly walked into her dentist's office. She recovered quickly and, within a few days, was back to herself. And she made herself a little cheat sheet for any future appointments.

HOW-TO FOR YOU

When scary doctor visits loom, your child may benefit from some of
the following practices.

⁑ Ask and Answer Questions

Clear information is a comfort and a way to strengthen the
imagery experience. Brainstorm together and make a list of
questions that your child has about the doctor visit. Answer
whatever questions you can. Gather additional information
if necessary. Your child can then rehearse more accurately
what will happen.

⁑ Create a Sense of Control

Determine what your child can actually control. Perhaps
not the procedure itself—or the fact that it will happen—but
he may have some say about the timing, where to celebrate
afterward, or what reward he can receive for cooperation.

⁑ Use a Practice Metaphor

Remind your child that he once had to practice to learn to
do things like tying his shoes, riding a bike, and reading.

Use a simple script: "To do well at a game, the team needs
to practice. The more they practice, the better they get. It's
the same for your doctor's visit." Try different approaches
until he sees the connection.

⁑ Visualize a Successful Outcome

Practicing a positive outcome before any procedure will
decrease fear. Have your child imagine being in his Special Place, surrounded by favorite animals and people. Ask
him to summon his *Bravery*. Suggest that the visit will go
extremely well and how proud he'll feel walking out of the

doctor's office. Evoke all his senses, so that the future experience is as real as possible. What is he wearing? What sounds does he hear on the street? What does the air feel like? What do you say to him afterward? This will strengthen his vision about being on the other side of the scary event.

▓ Create a Body Anchor

While your child is relaxed, ask him to tap gently on an easy-to-reach part of his body, such as his wrist or arm. Suggest that whenever he taps that spot, he will immediately be in a deep relaxed state, that he'll be confident and brave, knowing he can handle whatever is expected. Younger children may prefer holding a cherished toy. Remind him to do this when he arrives at the doctor's to ready himself for the procedure.

▓ Use Music

If you don't have much time to prepare, bring along a soothing soundtrack to use for general relaxation at the time of the procedure. He can listen to one of my recorded CDs or one of his other favorites.

Earthquakes, Floods, Terrorist Attacks, and More

Fear of Disasters

Slate was a sensitive and talented ten-year-old, who liked to draw and daydream. Then a major earthquake shook his world. He became afraid of being alone, even of going to the bathroom and sleeping by himself. Unlike other kids, who returned to normal activities within weeks of this frightening event, Slate's anxieties escalated to fears of noise from fans and dryers, lightning and thunder, and the possibility of his house burning down. An earlier unease with dogs returned. Previous minor behaviors—nail biting, anger, conflicts with siblings—became more intense. All this after only forty-five seconds of shaking!

Natural disasters are hard on everyone. Whether earthquakes, hurricanes, wildfires, tornados, tsunamis, or floods, nature always seems to be flexing her muscles in ways that spell disaster for some community. With easy access to TV news and its repeated, graphic content, the visual impact of faraway disasters can also traumatize or affect children deeply. As can witnessing or experiencing other calamities, like riots, community violence, and acts of terror. One seven-year-old, upon hearing about a large riot, went into his backyard and found a big stick to protect his family from the "bad men." An eleven-year-old who had seen violence on TV urged his mother to buy a gun. For weeks he slept on the floor next to the wall to protect himself from the possibility of bullets.

Children's emotional reactions vary in character and severity and are determined by age, temperament and personality, previous experiences, and the immediacy of the disaster. These reactions can include intense grieving, feelings of loss of control and stability, and practical concerns about safety, food, and clothing. Recurring nightmares are common, as are physical symptoms (headaches, stomachaches, poor or voracious appetite), behavioral changes (anger, withdrawal, restlessness, regression), and difficulty being alone or concentrating.

Most kids are able to resolve their feelings within six to eight weeks, and that time can be shortened with knowledgeable help. However, for children with preexisting or unresolved fears, reactions can last much longer. They are the ones, like Slate, who find their way to my office.

What most helped Slate was combining imagery with art. He developed a weekly routine of coming into my therapy playroom and drawing his fears, then having a dragon puppet symbolically eat them to make them disappear.

Bring the Safe Future into Now: To start Slate thinking about the possibility of recovery, I asked what life would be like when he did feel safe. If he could imagine where he would like to go or be (a safe place), then we could deal with any obstacles to getting there.

Hearts and Guts Know the Truth: After closing his eyes and focusing on his Balloon Breath, Slate consulted with the wisdom of Heart and Belly feelings. "My world will be peaceful again," he reported. "I won't be afraid of the earth exploding. I'll be able to sleep. I won't get that tight feeling in my chest. I'll be calm."

QUICK TIP! **Bring In the Senses**

Have your child imagine not only how it "feels" to be safe, but what it looks like, what sounds she hears, and what smells she detects. Evoking as many senses as possible will make the experience seem realer.

Record a Tape or CD: With the information Slate provided, we created a personalized safety imagery that helped him develop confidence and recover spontaneity. We used his favorite colors to relax his body, then had him imagine golden sunlight melting his fears and bringing him power and strength. Slate practiced every night. The repetition of positive images was just what he needed to regain his trust in a more secure world. Although he had a short attention span, he requested adding to the previous week's story. So I led him to a magical land where he could feel safe at all times. Protective Animal Friends brought him Gifts to help visualize doing the things he used to do—sleeping alone and playing and laughing with his friends. These longer, elaborated tapes increased the complexity of the message, allowing him to "catch" different concepts on different nights. He loved the personal touch of his name appearing throughout the imagery.

Reassurance Is Good—and So Are Warm Hands: Because Slate had such a fragile temperament, I was extra soothing and reassuring. I also used energy work to calm him. After I centered myself, I pictured him feeling safe and imagined loving energy pouring from my heart down through my arms into my hands. Then I placed my hands on Slate's shirt at his lower back. He felt the warmth from the energy flowing. It relaxed him and distracted him from his fears of catastrophe. Later, I taught him how to do the same for himself, but with his hands on his stomach.

Use a Rainbow for Protection: Slate loved color, so it was not surprising that he chose to breathe in a whole rainbow to feel safe. As the colors came into the top of his head and slowly filtered down through his body, they helped him release fears, worries, and anger about the earthquake. I suggested that he could replace any negative feelings by breathing in positive images of peace, calmness, and love.

Once the rainbow light filled him, I encouraged Slate to extend it past his body—six inches, one foot, then three. He imagined himself inside a giant safe cocoon. He sealed it with silver, allowing only good to come through, deflecting scary or bad thoughts. Armed with his own shield, Slate moved forward.

Backtrack Alert

You might wonder if allowing Slate to create an imaginary protective shell gave him a false sense of security. In case of disasters, we rarely have much control over the outcome. But with these new skills, Slate could think more clearly and make healthier decisions. To function in his everyday life, he needed to overcome his trauma fears. Giving him life-affirming tools was a step in that direction. Of course, should another natural disaster hit, Slate would probably regress. Anyone would. But he would be better prepared to bounce back more quickly.

Develop Affirmations: Slate learned the power of positive self-talk, repeating one or several of these affirmations throughout the day:

- I can breathe in calm and peace.
- If there's an earthquake, I know how to make myself safe.
- If there is lightning (or thunder), I am safe.
- I am taken care of.
- No matter what happens around me, I am safe.

Create the Butterfly of Transformation: Slate diligently developed his protective cocoon. He practiced two to three times a day, three to five minutes each session. After a few months, he was able to imagine turning into a butterfly as all the colors swirled around him. He had rainbow wings, flew freely, and felt nothing could harm him. It was a revelation when he realized how much he had changed, that he had let go of his fears of imminent danger and could feel his happy spirit again.

HOW-TO FOR YOU

Children can grow stronger after traumatic situations. Whatever calamity your child has been exposed to, imagination techniques can not only help her overcome that experience, but also prepare her to react more confidently and recover more quickly if another disaster should occur.

⬢ Make the Future Now

Have your child visualize that it's two weeks, two months, or a year after she's achieved her goal of feeling safe from disaster. Looking back as if her fear is far in the past will strengthen her vision for reaching her goal.

⬢ Create a Recording

Use your child's dream of safety to create a recorded imagery she can use on her own. Guide her into deep relaxation and incorporate suggestions about feeling calm and safe, trusting that help is available, and developing her own ability to handle whatever she's faced with. Or you can use the Feeling Safe guided journey at the end of this chapter. The freedom to listen whenever she wants can give her a bit more control in a chaotic world.

Offer Loving Touch

Disasters trigger panic, both in the moment and the aftermath. And a panicked person can't think straight. Tapping into Energy can restore balance and release bottled tensions. You can do Energy healing for your child to help her feel more secure, and then teach her to do it for herself.

Just center yourself and imagine the love you feel for your child spreading from your Heart into your hands. Place them on her mid or lower back and send her thoughts of love and safety. Now imagine pulling the panic feelings into your palms and releasing them into the atmosphere through the back of your hands. See how she feels.

Practice Affirmations

Use sentences that reinforce the desired goal. Your child can start with: "Each day I feel safer and more comfortable in my room alone." Then try: "I feel safe and comfortable reading in my room alone." Now try the same two-step with ". . . at school" or ". . . at the mall." Slowly adapt the affirmation to her particular routines and anxieties. The idea is to be positive and move, step by step, toward her final affirmation: "I feel safe and comfortable in the world around me."

Pick an Animal to Symbolize Success

Invite an Animal Friend to come support your child. A courageous lion, a soaring eagle, a snake shedding its old skin, or like

Slate, a butterfly symbolizing transformation from fearful to free. Have her ask it to appear when she's at or near her goal.

Why Do People Die, and Is It Going to Happen to Me?

Fear of Dying

"I'm afraid I'm going to die." Looking up with pools of indigo eyes, five-year-old Roxie announced this the first time we met. I knew about Roxie's fear from my session with her parents, but had not expected her to be so honest and vulnerable in our first encounter. Roxie's fear of dying affected all aspects of her life. "I'm afraid if I swallow a chocolate, I will choke. I'm afraid if I touch a leaf, I'm going to be poisoned." And most disturbingly, "I'm afraid if I see a bee, it's going to fly into my ear and eat my brain."

Few fears surpass that of dying. We don't like to think about it, especially in relation to ourselves. Some people have strong spiritual or religious beliefs in an afterlife, Heaven, or reincarnation, which may offer comfort. Others are not so sure and want scientific proof. No matter what families believe, children have difficulty coming to terms with the finality of death. The thought of being separated from those they love can be dreadful. So we often try to protect them from the notion of death. But as Roxie taught her parents, that doesn't always work.

Roxie was from a gentle, wonderful family. There were no traumas, shocks, or illnesses to cause such a big fear. But one summer day, walking in the country with her parents, she came upon a small dead rabbit. She tried to process the image in her young mind, but couldn't. A flood of questions followed. She asked what happens when a person dies, then went through a list of everyone she knew, wanting to know, one by one, if each would die.

Although these kinds of questions are expected when a child loses a close friend or family member, Roxie had not yet experienced death up close—no pets, family, or friends. It was this first exposure to death that set Roxie's mind going.

Her parents explained what they believed—that the rabbit was in "Heaven up in the clouds." They stressed that, since it likely had been ill, it was better off there. This gave her temporary comfort. Months later, Roxie returned to the same countryside. Within a week, she had trouble sleeping, developed dark circles under her eyes, her color faded, and her heart raced. Roxie's fear was so huge, she cried, "I don't want to die!"

Although her parents reassured her that she was young and healthy, that dying wasn't in the picture for a long time, the fears wouldn't dissipate—not even when she was safely back home. Roxie's anxiety created such walloping stomach pain, her family ended up in the emergency room late one night. After three hours of evaluation, including invasive blood and urine tests, nothing physical was found. That's when her pediatrician referred them to me.

Draw a "Body Picture" to Identify Feelings: Because Roxie was so young, and in a near panic state, I took the first step and drew an outline of her body. I asked her to close her eyes and look inside to imagine where her fearful parts were. "What color and shape are they? What picture do they create?"

Give Feelings Shape and Color: Roxie identified her worried feelings as simple large square shapes. *Fear* was black and over her heart; *Worry* was purple in her legs. To help her focus on the positive feelings that could help her, we added *Brave* (a blue circle in her brain) and *Happy* (two pink circles, one in each shoulder). Roxie witnessed her own power as she breathed Brave Blue into Black Fear. Her worries began to fade.

Feelings Often Have Stories: Roxie described how Brave was like a teenager, more grown-up than she was. Sometimes it was in her brain, other times in her heart. Fear was like a baby, sometimes in her chest as a big square, other times in her belly as a small circle. When she breathed in Brave Blue, the scared baby got a bottle and was soothed.

Use Physical Gestures: What reassured Roxie most was touching her Heart center (the center of her chest at heart level) with her hand while doing her Balloon Breath. The physical gesture made her self-comfort more powerful, and she became calm enough to consider creating a safe place.

Find Comfort in Your Special Place: Roxie's was inside her favorite imaginary mode of transport—a powerful black train, with inviting red seats and a TV—traveling happily with her family to a nearby town. She put orange light around the train to shield herself and her loved ones, but by the time she drew the picture, her protection colors turned pink and blue.

Backtrack Alert

There's no need to be concerned if your child says one thing during her imagery experience, and does another later. She may change the shape, place, and color of her feelings. What is important is that she be aware of them and notice where they are in her "body/mind." It's the process that's key.

Choose Favorite Tools: After practicing each skill twice, Roxie chose what felt best. Mom reported on progress: "She likes to breathe deeply to calm herself, and she derives great comfort by looking at the drawing of the safe train." Once Roxie was able to quell her fears around the subject of death, her parents were able to use the experience to share with her their views on dying and the circle of life.

Just two months later, Roxie's parents noticed real improvement. "She's herself again, more relaxed, joking, and happy. If any little fears come up, she manages them. She's sleeping great—eleven to twelve hours a night—and now has a more realistic view of death."

HOW-TO FOR YOU

As we have seen, Roxie learned to be more comfortable around the big issue of dying. Your child can, too.

⠿ Identify Feelings with a "Body Picture"
Use an 11-by-17-inch piece of paper, tape two pieces of poster-size paper together, or trace your child's body on butcher paper. Older kids can draw for themselves. Then have him close his eyes, imagine where his fears about death or dying are located in his body, and add them to his Body Picture drawing.

⠿ Take Advantage of the Colors and Shapes of Feelings
Have your child imagine what color and shape his fearful and brave parts are. Help him practice breathing the Brave color into his Fear of Death. Notice what happens. Play with other positive and negative feelings this way.

⠿ Talk to Your Feelings
Have your child ask his Fear of Death to reveal its story. Adjust the language based on his age.

1 What would be helpful to be aware of or understand?
2 What do I have to do differently to release my fear?
3 How can I make my brave part stronger?
4 How can I make confidence bigger?
5 What help do I need from my parents?

⦂ Take Time to Talk

Whenever the subject of death comes up in any form, from a scene on TV to the death of a neighbor or pet, you can use it as a launching pad for a talk about your views on death, dying, and the life cycle. These are hard concepts for children to grasp, whether they have experienced a death or not. Don't be surprised if you have the same conversation more than once.

⦂ Practice "Good Health" Homework

Take five to ten minutes a few times a day to have your child practice whichever Tools feel right to him. Once he moves past his fear of death or dying, the Tools will keep him on a healthy healing track.

⦂ Distinguish Between Fear and Loss

If your child's fear of death stems from an actual death in his life, then grief is fueling his fear. Chapter 9 is dedicated to coping with loss. Will and Heather's stories, and the How-To's that follow, will help you address his underlying sorrow. Grief and fear are a painful partnership, as one can often impersonate the other. You will need to attend to each feeling as it shows up. And be patient. It takes time for Hearts to heal.

Feeling Safe
A Guided Imagery Script

No matter the nature of your child's fear—abandonment, change, the unknown, doctors, disasters, or dying—the underlying need is to feel safe. The following journey is designed to foster a core sense of safety and a trust that he or she can handle whatever life may bring.

Be aware of the air going into your nose, down into your belly, and then out again through your nose. Let yourself find a comfortable rhythm breathing in and out slowly—one . . . two . . . three . . . Now, be aware of your chest and your heart. Picture your heart in the middle of your chest. As you breathe in and out, imagine a spark of light inside it. It may be as small as a dot—or it may already be large. It may be white, or pink, or green, or any color you like. Imagine this dot of light expanding with every slow breath you take, like a kernel of growing love and hope. Let it bring security and comfort to melt away fears and worries, filling your Heart and chest like a rippling rainbow.

Continue to breathe slowly as light gently spreads its warmth through your body, filling you with peace and calm. You have all the time you need. When this light of safety fills your whole body, imagine its protection spreading six inches past your skin. Very good. Notice if your protective light changes as it grows—out one foot, two feet, three feet. It surrounds all of you—front, back, top, bottom, sideways—like being in a protective egg.

Now, picture putting a special seal around your safety light. It may be gold, silver, copper, or any other color. Inside you are safe and secure; nothing bad can come in. Only good. You are protected by your bubble of safety light. Anything harmful bounces off—back to where it came from.

Whenever you're in need, help is always available . . . from your inner protector, your parents, a trusted adult, or a friend. You will know whom to call. You will know when you can take care of things yourself and when to ask for aid.

Each morning when you wake up, start your day safe and secure. Take a few minutes to relax and connect with your Heart, and allow your protective light to expand. You can do this in the morning, afternoon, or at night—anytime you'd like to melt away fears or worries. Anytime you'd like to feel safer and more secure. And each time you practice, it gets easier and easier to connect to your inner protector. You are safe.

Bedtime

**If you believe you're
already sleeping, you'll be
asleep in a minute.**
—*Sophie, age eight*

Getting a Good Night's Sleep and Overcoming Bed-Wetting

★ t's the end of the day. You're tired. The children have finally gone to bed, and you're looking forward to some peace, or maybe private time with your partner. Suddenly you see your five-year-old creeping out of bed. Or your preteen charges into the room insisting she can't shut her eyes; she's worried about an exam, a fight with a friend, her hair. Worse yet, you're already asleep, and your eight-year-old starts wailing. His bed is soaked . . . again. You almost start wailing yourself.

Children's sleep problems are all too frequent; 30 to 69 percent of kids experience a disorder at some point. Over one third of all parents nationwide report their children have a hard time getting out of bed, are restless sleepers, or awaken grouchy.[1] Bed-wetting is another common reason kids wake up. And when your child is up at night, odds are you can't sleep either.

Sound sleep is critical for everyone's physical and emotional well-being. When it's disrupted, bodies are stressed and immune systems weaken, making us vulnerable to infection. Sleeplessness affects mood, memory, and learning, too. Sleep-deprived kids may be aggressive, sluggish, or overactive. In time, depression can set in. Sleeplessness creates not only a cranky and poorly performing student at school, but also an unhappy, unhealthy child at home.[2]

With inadequate sleep, the brain's emotional centers overreact to negative experiences, shutting down the area that keeps emotions under control (*prefrontal cortex*), and reverting to more primitive responses.[3] So when your child snaps at you after a restless night, there's good reason. And if you've been up for hours with your nightmare-plagued daughter, you just might snap back.

It's a vicious cycle. Kids who get less sleep one night have more trouble drifting off the next. Jonah, age seven, couldn't get a good night's rest because he feared little green men were attacking his brain when he slept. One carried a long gun with a poison green tip. He'd shoot it and ruin Jonah's dreams. Poor Jonah didn't stand a chance. Each sleepless night increased his belief in the creature's power; it became increasingly difficult for him to conceive of a good night's sleep.

Adequate sleep prepares our kids for doing their best physically, emotionally, and academically. They resist illnesses, have more energy, exhibit nicer moods, and get along better with friends and family. Well-slept children also pay better attention at school, generate more creative ideas, and solve problems more easily.[4]

How much sleep is enough? That depends on your child. Age and development certainly affect sleep requirements—a four-year-old may need twelve hours while a twelve-year-old does well on nine—but so does individual constitution.[5] One tween complained she was sent to bed at a "reasonable" time all through elementary school. But twelve hours was more sleep than her body needed. She'd lie in bed for hours, mind racing, or she'd read by flashlight under the covers until she drifted off. She wound up getting about eight hours a night—perfect for her.

What constitutes a sleep problem also varies from home to home and culture to culture. In many families, children sleep in their own beds or rooms; crawling in with Mom and Dad for any reason is discouraged. Other homes have a "family bed," and it's normal for kids to pile in. Cosleeping is quite common: 35 to 55 percent of preschoolers and 10 to 23 percent of school-aged children sleep with their parents.[6] There are, of course, many families in the middle: kids cuddle in their parents' big bed but are carried to their own just before or once they fall asleep. Be aware that if your child is falling asleep with you—either in your room or in his—he may not be learning to sleep on his own. How your family handles sleeping arrangements is up to you—as long as your children are, in fact, sleeping.

If your child is not, the Nine Tools can help. The same young imagination that creates dramatic doubts before bedtime can also learn to let go of the day's worries. Imagery can teach your child to put himself to sleep on his own. It can also train a sound sleeper to awaken at the sensation of a full bladder instead of a wet bed. These skills are so automatic we ignore them—until they don't work. Your child's imagination can provide a creative, positive, and efficient route to sleep success.

In this chapter we explore three of the most common bedtime dilemmas:

- Trouble falling asleep.
- Trouble staying asleep.
- Trouble keeping a dry bed.

Help . . . I Can't Fall Asleep!

How to Get a Good Night's Rest

At eight, Sophie was an exhausted second grader. Tossing and turning, she couldn't settle her body and mind until after 11:00 p.m. Waking Sophie was torture. She was short-tempered all day. Her mom tried warm baths, herbal tea, eliminating sugar and soda, even homeopathic remedies to help Sophie fall asleep. Nothing worked. Finally, her pediatrician suggested she come to me.

Trouble falling asleep is the most common sleep complaint I hear. Younger kids often resist bedtime out of fear of being alone or separating from their parents. Older kids may be fixated on the day's upsetting events. Being overtired or overworried are common causes of sleeplessness, as are fears of bad dreams, nightmares, or dark, imagined creatures. Many children simply never developed the skills to put themselves to sleep.

Sophie knew exactly what her problem was. "I can't turn off my brain," she said. At bedtime, "stuff comes spilling out," or some big life question would grab her attention. Sophie had never been a good sleeper, and she didn't realize that other kids fell asleep easily. Thank goodness once she finally did fall asleep, she was out for the night.

Be Prepared for Dark Thoughts: I asked Sophie to describe what her life was like now. She snatched my markers and drew herself without detail, floating in space in the land of "No Love." "All the flowers are dead," she explained. "The grass is dark, and the worst part is, it's raining." Bleak thoughts are common among sleepless kids; it's not just parents who are stressed.

Visualize Transformation: Then I asked Sophie how her life would be different when she could fall asleep easily. I wanted to see if she could imagine the possibility of sleep. Her drawing took us into the land of "Love." The sun was shining, clouds were white, and everything was growing. Sophie drew herself in great detail as a princess. That she could picture a life in which she slept peacefully was a positive sign. It meant our work toward her goal could start immediately.

Backtrack Alert

Sometimes a kid cannot imagine sleeping peacefully. If this is the case, find something positive he *can* imagine. Can he envision sleeping easily in five months? A year? As a grown-up? Start there and gently move forward. Say, "So, when you're a dad like me, you'll be able to fall asleep quickly? What's going to help you do that?" Incorporate whatever your child tells you into his new "falling asleep easily" plan. Be patient; learning these skills doesn't happen overnight.

Imagine Sleeping Effortlessly: Sophie also verbalized what her life might be like when she could fall asleep easily: She'd feel more relaxed and refreshed. The dark circles under her eyes and her crabbiness would vanish. Most of all, she'd feel "really, really happy inside" and "very proud" of herself. Her ability to visualize her goal, and express in words her desire for success, set the tone for what followed.

Face Obstacles: Our next step was to address what specifically was keeping Sophie from sleeping. "Scared feelings, worries, all the bad things creeping me out," she said. I asked what she needed to clean out these dark thoughts, and suggested she close her eyes to better see her inner TV screen. Sophie imagined washing her negative mind with colorful bubbles that turned the blackness into shiny gold pearls. She rehearsed this image in my office and, when she was comfortable, practiced at home.

Share Your Troubles: We needed to help Sophie let go of bedtime worries so she could relax. Her parents agreed to hear her woes each night as they tucked her in. If they were unavailable, a trusted babysitter would do. This became a comforting nightly ritual.

Welcome Wizards Bearing Gifts: Next, we invited a Wizard to join us. Sophie imagined Hermione (à la *Harry Potter*) appearing in a flowing violet skirt, bright pink blouse, and gold crown. I suggested that her Wizard might have a Gift to help her sleep. Almost immediately, she envisioned Hermione bringing medicine—berries from a magical bush. Hermione instructed Sophie to picture chewing the blueberries slowly, one by one, allowing her body to rest deeply. She left Sophie with this wise advice: "If you believe you're already sleeping, you'll be asleep in a minute."

Accept the Learning Curve: Sophie progressed as expected. She would have a few good weeks, then trouble for the next two. But this dance of two steps forward, one back, is the natural learning curve for new behavior. By accepting this pattern as normal, her parents stayed calm on the harder nights. And as sleeping slowly became easier, Sophie's daytime attitude improved.

Seal the Deal with a Blanket of Sleep: After a few months, one final session completed our process. Sophie imagined herself in bed. "What's the coziest picture you can conjure?" I asked. She invented a blanket of sleep washing over her as she drifted off effortlessly. It's an accessible and comforting image, adding a sense of nurturing and security. She included Hermione, who offered support and waved her magic wand to create a cuddly angel bear that kept Sophie safe and snug.

Before she left, Sophie created her own easy bedtime hints—not a recap of our work together but additional reminders from her wise self to her bedtime self.

HOW-TO FOR YOU

You can apply what Sophie learned about putting herself to sleep to help your child have a good night's rest. Try these . . .

✳ Follow a Predictable Sleep Ritual

Rituals provide a sense of safety and may cue your child that it's bedtime. A warm bath, story time or reading for fifteen minutes, listening to soft music or a relaxation CD can lull a child to sleep.

✳ Help Him Imagine Sleeping Peacefully

Ask, "What's your life going to look like when you fall asleep easily on your own?" If he has trouble, casually offer ideas: "I wonder if you'll feel happy when you've learned to fall asleep easily. Maybe you'll have more energy for sports." Or, "Perhaps waking up will be easier."

❖ Give Woes Their Due

Invite your child to share his daily difficulties and worries. Say, "I'd like to hear about your troubles. Let's take five or ten minutes before you let them go for today and allow yourself to fall asleep." Set a timer if necessary. If there are leftover woes, suggest he imagine putting them in a colored balloon and letting them drift off. Assure him that if they return tomorrow, you will listen some more.

❖ Call In the Guides

Have him ask for one of his inner guides to show up. It might be an Animal Friend or Wizard. See what Gifts or advice they provide. Sleep potions and magic dreaming dust are common offerings, but your child may come up with something completely different, like Sophie's magical berries.

❖ Offer Comfort

In a soothing tone remind him, "You are safe. We will protect you so nothing hurts you. You'll be comfy in your bed all night." Don't underestimate the power of reassurance. Your child might not show it, but your every word penetrates.

❖ Be Realistic

Let your child know that it's natural to occasionally have trouble falling asleep. Worrying about it just makes matters worse. Assure him that lying quietly can be restful and restorative.

❖ Use "Blanket of Sleep" Imagery

If he still needs assistance, read or record the "Good Sleep Meditation" at the end of this chapter. Add his favorite images to suit him; he can listen while drifting off to sleep.

❖ Accept the Process

Your child has well-worn habits; be patient. It can take two to six months to see lasting change. Notice—and celebrate—small improvements such as fewer trips out of bed and quicker doze times. Each one leads toward the final goal of falling asleep easily.

Trouble in Snooze Town

How to Return to Sleep

Every night, several times a night, seven-year-old Nicole would come running into her parents' room, and every night, several times a night, her dad would take her back and sit with her until she returned to sleep. Dad could appreciate Nicole's night fears because he had had the same experience as a youngster. But when he traveled and couldn't keep her company, she fell apart.

According to Mom, Nicole had "horrible sleeping habits" from the start and slept with her parents until she was three. The situation eased once she began sharing a room with her sister. When the family moved, her parents thought it was the perfect time for Nicole to try her own room. But she was terrified without her sister or father there when she awoke. It didn't matter that she was safe; Nicole couldn't soothe herself back to sleep alone. Mom was fed up, and everyone was worn out. Nicole clearly needed to develop skills for putting herself back to bed.

All children awaken briefly at night, sometimes repeatedly, owing to bad dreams, toilet needs, or disturbances in the lighter sleep cycles.[7] Most quickly return to sleep. But when a child is unable to calm himself or to feel safe enough to release his body, he won't fall back asleep. And if parents consistently "help" by offering company until he nods off, that child is more likely to have difficulty learning new sleep habits.

Nicole had a whole list of anxieties about sleeping and waking alone. She was afraid that when she awoke in her empty room, the world might blow up, a comet might hit the house, the bogeyman might arrive, a thief might break in, or monsters might suffocate her. And when she was able to put herself back to sleep, she'd reawaken with nightmares. She couldn't accept her mom's explanation that dreams weren't real.

Add Heart Light for Insurance: To help Nicole feel connected to her parents, I suggested she imagine sending love from her heart to theirs on a colored beam of light. As her parents received her love, they sent theirs back. That way, Nicole felt close to them but didn't have to be in their bedroom. She chose a pink love-beam, Mom chose yellow, and Dad blue. We practiced with Mom in my office, then in the waiting room, and finally they practiced at home.

Find Your Own Dream Space: For kids who can't imagine feeling safe enough to fall back asleep, it's important to create an inner sanctuary during the day. I asked Nicole to picture a spot where she felt protected. She created a "dream place" in the sky where a rainbow escalator led up to a big cloud and turned into a slide going down. I suggested she use that image at night as she fell asleep and again if she awakened.

Ms. Emerald and the White Sleeping Powder: For added support, I wondered if a special Animal Friend might come to Nicole's dream place. Ms. Emerald appeared—a snow-white Unicorn with a rainbow horn and golden mane and tail. Not surprisingly, her name came from her bright green eyes. She lived on top of the clouds.

Ms. Emerald offered Nicole a Gift to help with this "wake up in the night" problem: white sleeping powder in a green perfume jar. "You sprinkle it on your head, and you say 'falling asleep,' and then you sleep for the whole night." How often should they meet? Nicole's message was clear: "Every single, pingle, wingle, tingle night because she keeps my sleeping powder."

QUICK TIP! **Things Don't Always Make Sense**

Kids aren't always consistent. First Ms. Emerald gives Nicole sleep medicine to use on her own, then she says she needs to provide it. That's okay. The image doesn't have to be consistent, just real and alive for your child.

Take a Magic Carpet Ride: I wanted Nicole to have a variety of options in case some Tools didn't always work. While visiting her dream place, I asked Nicole to fashion a vehicle that would take her to a castle. Nicole used pink, lemon, lime, turquoise, and fuchsia to create a magic carpet where she relaxed as she floated. An animal buddy, Bird, flew alongside, adding an "all-around good feeling."

Visit a Magic Castle for Gifts: They arrived safely at a striped palace through a sparkling Welcome door. Here Nicole received three Gifts to help her return to sleep: a shiny gold crown that made her feel more powerful, a silver drum that created rain—she loved listening to its sound as she drifted off—and a box with rainbows shooting out of it that sprinkled dust on Nicole and helped her fall back asleep. "It just settles me," she explained.

Use Imagination to Control Dreams: Nicole's scary dreams made it difficult for her to fall back asleep: she was on a roller coaster and fell into a pool of sharks; a vampire was trying to kill her; the world was dark and never sunny. I had her draw these dreams to work with their characters. In each situation, I suggested she ask her imagination to project a helpful image on an inner computer screen. Nicole envisioned swimming away from the sharks and her parents lifting her from the water. She imagined finding garlic bread and telling the vampire it was toast; when he ate it, he died. As for waking with the earth in darkness, Nicole pictured flipping a switch that turned the sunlight back on. Each exercise built her confidence and skill, so that eventually, upon awakening, she'd be able to transform her scary dreams into ones she could live with and, more importantly, sleep with.

Sandman Faces Off with Grumpy: After weeks of diligent practice, a part of Nicole still waffled on handling mid-night upsets. The Tools she had been learning so far often worked, but not all the time. So I introduced a new one, a variation on Talking to Toes, and asked her to go inside her body to see what feelings were blocking the way and what, or who, might help. Answers came in the form of two cartoon characters. Grumpy, who looked miserable, wore a green shirt and purple hat; he was determined to stay up and do whatever he wanted. Sandman was happy and upbeat. He had a black beard, wore hot pink, and carried a bag of sand. He sprinkled sand on Grumpy, which immediately put Grumpy to sleep. As he drifted off, Sandman reminded him that he could also have fun in his dreams. When Grumpy did awaken, he regretted his mischievous ways. He should have fallen back to sleep quickly all along and been less grumpy. By unconsciously giving voice to her ambivalence about bedtime, these images helped Nicole resolve her dilemma.

Backtrack Alert

Grumpy might seem to indicate Nicole's willfulness, but when kids insist on staying up, or they need another drink of water in the middle of the night, the delay tactics often protect them from their fears about getting back to sleep. Helping your child find his own solutions can resolve this problem.

When Nicole completed her work with me, she was doing great. Her Mom called a few months later to let me know she was now teaching her younger brother how to stay in *his* bed!

HOW-TO FOR YOU

Nicole was able to use her imagination to diffuse her anxiety about sleeping and waking alone. I hope her process inspires you to teach your sleepless child these skills. It's best to practice during the day when things are calm; learning new skills before bed can create pressure. But gentle bedtime reminders of what he's already learned can be welcome.

Connect Through Sending Loving Light

Have your child imagine his love for you, and yours for him, as two different colors. As he does his Balloon Breath, he sends his "love color" in a beam of light from his Heart to yours. At the same time he visualizes receiving your bright love in his Heart. This connection can help him feel more secure and less alone when he is trying to go back to sleep on his own.

Create an Ideal Sleep Space

Ask your child to imagine the best spot to sleep—where he will feel perfectly safe and protected. He can create any place and add anyone he wants there for support.

See Who Shows Up

Request one of the people or animals that live in his ideal sleep space to help him fall back asleep by giving a Gift or a message, or showing him something he never thought of before. He may receive special sleep medicine or his dream room may reveal hidden treasures.

Visit a Castle and Accept Its Gifts

Offer the possibility of being a guest in a magic castle—often kept for the very privileged. Let your child know that the Gift he receives there to help him fall back asleep will surely be special. A younger child might be particularly taken with this idea.

Take Charge of Dreams

During the day when all is safe, ask your child to imagine how he'd like his bad dream to end, or how he'd like to change it. Have him close his eyes and redo the dream to his liking. This will increase his confidence and is a start to gaining power over nightmares. Plant the idea that, with a little practice, he'll be able to do the same thing for himself if a bad dream wakes him.

Confront the Dark Side

As much as your child wants to fall asleep, a part of him might enjoy all the attention when he can't. That's normal. Ask him to close his eyes, look inside his body and brain, and imagine if there's a spot that actually lights up at the idea of staying awake. Invite him to ask that part, "What do I need to do to fall asleep on my own? What do I need to know to accept my ability to fall asleep?"

Brainstorm More Ideas

Ask your child to come up with his own "going back to sleep" ideas. Work together and keep a running list. For instance, part of his nightly routine could include requesting a good dream or an Animal Friend to stand guard.

Create Bedtime Speed Bumps

As your child learns to take himself back to bed, there will still be nights he calls for you, even if he's just slightly scared. Habits are hard to break. These are times when it's useful to have a reminder note of things he can do posted somewhere he can see them, such as on his bedroom door or yours. If he still comes to your bedroom, help him fall back asleep by sitting in his room and walking him through the Tools. Consider playing a CD to give his nervous mind a place to focus. Eventually he'll call on the Tools himself and let everyone get a good night's rest.

⠕ Respect Your Body's Needs

Sometimes you just need your sleep—perhaps you have an early meeting or you're just too exhausted to return him to bed. It's important to pick your battles. Sometimes the best thing for everyone is to go back to sleep as soon as possible, even if it means your child might temporarily regress. On those nights, go ahead and let him curl up in your room. You can revisit the Tools tomorrow.

Oh No, Wet Bed Again!

How to Keep Dry at Night

Mornings were the real source of stress for ten-year-old Kyle. Every night he'd go to sleep hoping for a dry bed, and every morning he'd awaken to discover soaked sheets. He was so embarrassed. Try as he might, this bright, athletic boy could not wake up in the middle of the night. He often dreamt that he was on the toilet, but he just peed in his sleep. The alarm his parents tried—the one that sounds when a drop of urine hits—woke everyone but him. The medication that was meant to shut down urine production at night didn't work. Nor could Kyle avoid drinking at night; he took karate two evenings a week and needed to quench his thirst. His parents were exhausted from all the struggle and effort, and they suffered over his suffering. They also felt responsible—and a tad guilty—since both had been bed-wetters as children. However, their major concern was to prevent Kyle from being teased when he went to sleepaway camp that summer.

Bed-wetting is common. Up to 20 percent of five-year-olds wet the bed, as do 10 percent of seven-year-olds and 3 percent of ten-year-olds. Five to seven million kids in the United States are affected. Some do it every night; others are more sporadic. Most kids outgrow it.[8]

Although bed-wetting is considered normal through age four, many pediatricians don't worry about it until age seven.[9] Many developmental issues can contribute to a wet bed, such as bladder size, insufficient hormones to decrease urine production at night, or a nervous system with an underdeveloped "wake up and pee" signal. And bed-wetting does run in families. If one parent did it, a child has a 43 percent chance of doing it, too.[10]

Even a normally "dry" kid can be affected by life's pressures and insecurities and start wetting the bed. In addition to common medical causes—urinary tract infections or pressure from constipation—stress, emotional upsets, and anxiety can contribute to new or renewed bed-wetting. So can a recent move, a new baby, death of a pet or loved one, or increased marital stress.[11]

If a child is wetting the bed, and it's bothering her—regardless of age or history—it should be addressed. The guilt, shame, embarrassment, anxiety, low self-esteem, and anger that commonly accompany bed-wetting can cause emotional trauma. Families suffer, too. Parents like Kyle's will try anything: limiting drinks after dinner, using medications, taking the child to the bathroom before he or she goes to sleep. But the wetness seems to come just when they leave. They end up exhausted and frustrated, struggling with their own embarrassment, anger, and helplessness, which can, inadvertently, make their child feel worse.

Fortunately, imagery is especially successful in controlling bed-wetting.[12] I have long used it, and the mind-body connection, to teach children to send messages from the bladder to the brain and back again so they awaken when the bladder is nearly full. They also strengthen it to hold more urine. By learning to relax deeply, turn inward, and listen to what their bodies truly need, children discover their unique path to a dry bed.

When I first met Kyle, he was on the last leg of a long journey to stay dry. He'd already conquered wetting during the day, but the nights still bothered him. During sleepovers, he stayed up as late as possible to hide in the bathroom and don his Pull-Ups. Then he woke before his friends to slip off the wet diaper in the morning. Although camp was six months away, Kyle felt pressure to perform, which only made matters worse.

Let Go of Personal Pressure: I told Kyle that if he hoped to succeed, he had to forget the deadline, just stay in the moment, do the best he could, and let go of the outcome. His first step was to calm down. Kyle learned to use the Balloon Breath and chose royal blue and gold, his favorite team's colors, to breathe in and help him relax.

Make Peace with a Younger You: Kyle also felt he was far too old to be wetting his bed. When I asked at what age he thought he should have stopped, he said, "By five, for sure." So we brought in the five-year-old version of Kyle for a conversation. Little Kyle was panicked and confused about why his bed-wetting was still happening. He felt it was his fault. I knew we had to calm this frightened, younger self before we could make progress. I encouraged older Kyle to reassure the little boy inside that he was going to be loved no matter what. They would surely get through this, and Big Kyle would take good care of him. This kindness seemed to be just what Little Kyle needed.

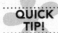

Talk to Your Little Kid

Talking to the little kid inside doesn't mean you're nutty. We talk to ourselves all the time when we are thinking. This is just a more directed way to gain clarity on a problem. Everyone has an inner child. You can help your youngster connect to hers; a ten-year-old can revisit her seven-year-old self, and a six-year-old can go back to age three. You can connect with your inner kid, too!

We then developed a multipronged approach to prepare Kyle for a dry night. He needed all the tools we could muster.

Beloved Old Dog and Helper Dude to the Rescue: When I suggested that Kyle ask for support from a guide, two assistants arrived: Cooper, Kyle's cherished canine who had died the year before, and "Happy Helper Dude." Cooper offered to bark and wake Kyle if he had to pee in the middle of the night, while Helper Dude was tiny enough to go inside his body and inspect the equipment.

Check Brain Switch: Helper Dude's job was to find and flip the switch in Kyle's brain that could turn off urine production at night. He floated around inside Kyle's head—past the front green area, which stored the things he loved to do, past his orange school section, across a yellow sports arena, and through the red love of family segment—until he finally reached his target. Helper Dude found the on-off switch in the very back of Kyle's mind. Luckily he carried a flashlight so he could locate the exact spot of this brain button.

Inspect the Bladder: When Helper Dude looked inside Kyle's bladder and urethra, they seemed to be in good shape. No holes or leaks, but the walls were thin. When he asked what color would help strengthen them, royal blue and gold came up again. He used these to coat the organs. Once the walls became strong and thick, Kyle envisioned his bladder having three knobs that kept urine from leaking out. One was located at the top center, while the other two flanked his urethra. They needed to be shut tight. Cooper helped by adding bricks and neon green sealant for extra protection.

QUICK TIP!   Draw a Picture of the Bladder

Most younger kids, and many older ones, have no idea what the bladder or urethra looks like, let alone what they do. Make a simple line drawing and give your child a straightforward explanation. This will give her a starting point for her own inner pictures.

Go to the Hall of Knowledge: To cover all bases, I urged Kyle to visit the "Hall of Knowledge," a place inside that holds all wisdom. Walking down pebble-dotted steps that took him deeper into this vast repository, I suggested that someone might meet him there. A "doctor" guide showed up. Since I was introduced to Kyle as Dr. Charlotte, I wasn't surprised that a doctor appeared in his imagination as well.

Add an Alarm: His doctor, aptly named Dr. P., suggested Kyle put an alarm clock on the top knob of his bladder to awaken him when his bladder was almost full. Kyle made sure to use Duracell batteries so his alarm wouldn't fail. Between Cooper's barking and the buzzer sounding, he would surely be roused.

Imagine Being Dry: Kyle's nightly homework was to imagine waking up dry, using all the richness his mind could offer: How he would feel. How the bed would smell. How happy he would be as he told his parents, "Dry again!" How proud they would be of him, and how proud he would be of himself. Then Kyle was to fast-forward to the future and imagine having been dry for six months.

Practice, Practice: He was to practice his stay-dry exercises before he went to sleep and also several times a day. Repetition deepened the imagery. It took only five minutes to "run" the whole routine, an internal maintenance check: Balloon Breath, check bladder and urethra for leaks or thin walls, fix any, check alarm clock for low batteries or malfunctions, and fix as necessary.

Positive Words Always Help: We also brainstormed a list of affirmations Kyle could use before bed. Each night, he chose three or four:

1 I deserve to be dry.
2 I have a dry bed.
3 I feel very proud now that I stay dry at night easily.
4 I wake up in the morning and my bed is dry.
5 My body and my bed are comfortable, and I stay dry.
6 If I must pee during the night, I wake up easily and go to the bathroom.

Reduce Pressure from Parents: I suggested that Kyle think about where he started—wet bed—to where he wanted to go—dry bed, and become aware of anything that was keeping him from his goal. He imagined walking along a path from wet to dry. Pressure from his mother was the obstacle. Her consistent encouragement felt like nagging, so instead of helping Kyle, her good intentions slowed his progress. Although I volunteered to help, Kyle took responsibility for speaking to her.

Be a Coach, Not a Badger

Pressure often produces panic. Of course you want to support your child, but this might be a time to step back. Ask her what she would like from you. Let her be in charge. Tell her you are there if she needs you, but don't ask how she did every day. Find out if she'd like your help, and if not, make a plan for her to practice on her own for a week or two. If it doesn't work out, you can always step gently back in.

Examine Your Beliefs: Kyle's progress was still inconsistent. Some weeks he'd be dry three days in a row, then wet for the next two. Or he'd have a solid dry spell of ten days followed by an awful week. Something seemed to be missing. I finally asked him to consider what he really believed about keeping a dry bed. Did he *hope* he could be dry, did he *believe* he could be dry, or did he *know* he could stay dry 100 percent of the time?

Kyle looked inside, and a big neon sign lit up: *Faith.* He needed more faith in himself. He asked where he could find faith. The answer was right inside him: "In my Heart." I wondered what this *Faith* looked like, and Kyle responded clearly. "It's invisible and feels warm and comfortable." I suggested he notice how he felt on any given day and whether his beliefs affected the next day's results. They did. Whenever he suspected a wet bed, that's what would happen, and when he expected to be dry, more often than not, he was. The days he felt like a lost cause were the ones he didn't bother to practice what he'd learned. And when he felt positive, he was more likely to follow his stay-dry plan.

This new awareness was powerful. Kyle reported a change from hoping he could be dry to actually knowing it. Soon, after consistent and loving inner work, he had just two wet mornings a month. And soon after that, he was . . . finally dry!

HOW-TO FOR YOU

Success often follows success. As your child brings her unique combination of self-caring rituals and stay-dry imagery techniques into her daily life, it will be possible to achieve her goal of a dry bed.

Give Permission to Release Pressure
Let your child know that bed-wetting is not her "fault," that kids eventually grow out of it, and that you are there for her.

Help Your Kids Imagine What Life Will Be Like Dry
A younger child might need some possibilities to choose from. Older ones might come up with their own ideas. Pick from the list below.

- Won't have so much to worry about.
- Won't have so much to hide.
- Won't have to sleep in a wet bed.
- Won't have to help Mom change the sheets.
- Won't have to wear Pull-Ups.
- Will be a lot easier to have sleepovers.
- Will feel proud of myself.

Scan the Body
Facilitate relaxing deeply with the Balloon Breath. Have her imagine going inside, inspecting the state of her bladder and urethra to see whether any damage or weakness might contribute to bed-wetting. Many children report that their bladder and/or urethra walls are thin, weak, or holey, making it difficult to hold urine at night.

✴ Use Color as a Healing Vehicle

Advise your child to ask her bladder or urethra what color would be helpful to breathe in to make it stronger and healthier or to patch any leaks. Use visualization to get her organs in tip-top shape.

✴ Install Internal Alarm Clock

Although your child is asking her bladder to hold urine all night, recommend she install an "alarm clock" as a backup. That way, if the bladder is full and about to "spill over," the alarm can awaken her in time.

✴ Meet Wise Counsel

Encourage her to ask for someone to show up and help. Use the bracketed script in the Good Sleep meditation (page 178) or your own words, including images and thoughts important to your child.

✴ Find Time to Practice

Propose she pick three times during the day to practice her "keep dry" exercises. Offer a few, such as on the way to school, or before homework or dinner.

✴ Use Positive Self-Talk

Suggest your child practice affirmations at bedtime. She can use Kyle's self-encouraging statements or create her own.

✴ Chart Stress and Progress

To bring awareness to the "keep dry" healing process, record your child's journey. Younger kids might enjoy earning stickers for a dry night; older kids might prefer handwritten positive comments, such as: "I'm proud of you," "You can do it," "Two in a row, that's great!" Some might write notes to themselves.

Blanket of Sleep
Good Sleep Meditation

The following guided imagery is effective for deep sleep. If your child has a problem with bed-wetting, add the script in brackets. Record this and have your child listen to it while drifting off to sleep, or read it to him before bedtime.

We're going to take some time now for you to relax and go very deep inside. To a place of peace, of quiet, and of [sweet dry] sleep. With each breath, your body becomes more and more relaxed. Imagine yourself lying down in a wonderful, comfortable bed. Perhaps it's like a fluffy white cloud that you can sink into. With each breath, your body sinks deeper and deeper into this soft, fluffy cloud.

Now picture a soft white light washing over your body, helping you to relax and putting you to sleep. As you breathe slowly, this lovely light melts through the top of your head, washes over your eyes and down your cheeks, relaxing you easily. You are drifting into sleep while this beautiful light continues to wash over your body. Each breath takes you deeper and deeper into sleep. The gentle light now moves through your neck and into your shoulders as it melts away all tension and worry.

It's time to let go . . . let go of all the thoughts of the day, of the week, of anything that's holding you back from sleep [and from staying dry]. As the light travels through your body, down your arms, into your chest, and around your heart, your heart opens and accepts healing light. Going deeper into sleep. Breathing into your belly, allowing the white light to blanket you. A blanket of sleep. As the soft relaxing light goes down into your legs, into your feet, and as you breathe, you float into safe sleep.

[Softly, quietly, you check in with that important part of you—your bladder. Gently ask it what it needs to keep you dry—tonight and every night—to wake you up when you need to use the bathroom. See how strong your bladder and urethra are. Notice if there are any leaks or holes that need to be fixed. Ask what color you can breathe in to help them grow stronger or seal any holes. Ask if any other body parts need love or acceptance. As you breathe, give your body whatever it needs.]

Now allow yourself to go back to a time when you fell into sleep as soon as your head touched the pillow [and you stayed dry until morning]. Back to this time when it was so easy to sleep [and stay dry]. Perhaps it was a long, long time ago. [Perhaps it hasn't happened yet.] But now, that time is here. You are peaceful, and happy, and easily asleep [and dry].

There may be caring animals around you, giving you comfort. Know you are totally safe as you go deeper and deeper into your sleep. Dreaming peaceful thoughts, precious thoughts.

Allow yourself to go deeper still until you meet a special being that has been waiting for you. A very wise and loving soul who takes your hand and leads you to even deeper sleep. Where you're safe [and dry] and comfortable—totally at peace.

[This wise being takes you deeper into the truth that awaits you, deep inside your heart, and shows you what you can do for yourself so that every night, and every morning, you are dry. You deserve to be dry. You are successful. And you drift off feeling good about taking care of yourself, your body, your mind, your heart—everything about you that keeps you dry.]

As you sleep, your heart expands. Love moves through your whole body. You drift into dreams. Wonderful dreams. Colors float around you. Smells of sleep comfort and surround you. Feel the softness of your blanket of sleep. Surprise yourself at how easy it is to sleep [and stay dry].

You stay in deep peaceful sleep for as long as your body desires. Any sounds or movements that you might hear or feel tell your body to sleep as long as you need to. You are protected. If you need to awaken, you will. [As soon as you need to use the bathroom, your inner alarm will tell you.] So you can just let go and sleep. As your body rests, all is good—as you sleep.

And each night as you lie in bed, sleep welcomes you and comes quickly. You fall asleep easily. You have peaceful and restful [dry] nights. You deserve this. As you accept that you deserve to sleep easily and peacefully, you sleep deeply [and stay dry].

CHAPTER 9

Why Does Everyone Keep Leaving?

Coping with Death, Divorce, and Other Losses

> If I'm sad, the sea lions make me smile. If I'm angry, Tiger shows me the place where I don't need to be. If I'm worried, Wizard tells me it's going to be okay in the future.
>
> —*Madison, age eleven*

★ riends move. Beloved pets die. Big sisters go to college. Parents separate and divorce. Grandparents pass away. Loss is an unfortunate fact of life. Everyone goes through it, some of us more than others. One young client had already survived her parents' divorce and the deaths of her grandmother and her favorite cat—all by the age of nine. "It's too bad that people that die are people we know," she observed philosophically, "and that people we know die."

Children form strong attachments. Any kind of abandonment—real or imagined—is painful to them. Someone who leaves, whether by choice or through accident or illness, is still someone leaving *them*—and with a hole in their lives. Whether your child is experiencing a death or a less permanent departure, loss brings grief. And a grieving child can break a parent's heart.

Grief is a dynamic process that presents us with four essential "tasks" in order to move forward: to accept the reality and finality of the loss, to experience its pain, to adjust to a life without our loved ones, and to find a new place for them in our hearts.[1] Grieving is individual and cannot always be predicted, and some losses are never fully reconciled. People mourn in their own time, and children will mourn differently depending on their age, personality, and maturity level. Some kids become angry, withdrawn, or distraught, like four-year-old Kenny. After his parents separated, he scribbled thick black marker over a drawing of a heart and announced, "My heart is dead." Others feel guilty or fearful. They believe a death was their fault or that they'll die now. They may also fear future losses. Aaron was just six when his mom died. He was afraid he wouldn't remember her and was jealous of his older sister, who had her longer.

Some kids grieve with their bodies—with aches, rashes, or nervous tics—or they regress or act out. Schoolwork suffers; sleeping and eating habits change. Harry, five, started gorging on junk food when his parents divorced, while Prudence, nine, stopped eating altogether. Then there are children who hide dramatic signs of grief; they may try to behave well or overachieve to counter their feelings of helplessness.

However your child reacts, remember that change and loss are frightening. These events tell him that life is unstable and out of his control. While you can't shield your child from loss, you can certainly arm him with healthy tools to soothe himself and face the challenges life inevitably brings.

Imagery uses a child's creativity to express his grief and adapt to loss. Consider Sabrina, who was four when her parents divorced. At ten, she still felt the old shock and hurt. She used her imagination to comfort her younger self—holding her in her lap, giving her love, and reassuring her that she'd done nothing wrong. This brought a new level of healing to "Little Sabrina"—and to Big Sabrina, as well. Six-year-old Malcolm cried every night after his grandpa died, until he imagined "PaPa" up in Heaven on big fluffy clouds, holding him in a big bear hug and saying, "Be happy. I'm happy now, too." And

Deborah, eleven, thought that after her mom's long illness, she was ready to release her. But when she died, Deb's heart shattered anyway. "What do I need to know to help me with my feelings about my mom's death?" she wrote in her journal. Her nondominant hand replied with a sober and honest answer: "If you love someone, you have to learn to let them go!" She reread these words every day for a year.

Letting go is not easy for anyone, but it's much harder for children. Let's look at how they can use the Nine Tools to work through three of the major losses life doles out:

- Parental divorce or separation
- The death of a pet
- The death of a loved one

These coping skills are easily transferred to other losses, great and small.

Divorce

How to Cope When Parents Split

When Madison's parents separated, she felt pressured to take sides. Her father wanted a divorce; her mother didn't. Both felt guilt and shame, which spilled on to their eleven-year-old. She began to gain weight, and her vivacious personality soured. She argued with her younger siblings and demanded attention. When her parents finally sought outside help, Madison had been crying and fighting for six months.

Divorce is an enormous loss for children and can have a life-long impact.[2] It's actually many losses rolled into one. The end of Mom and Dad living together and of the family as they've known it can also mean giving up a familiar house, local friends, and the consistency of the same bed each night. Divorce also breaks the predictability that children crave. They can feel their world is shattering. "But it's only a separation," say some parents. "We're not talking divorce yet." And some couples never will. But while the adults are working things out, the kids are bracing for the worst. It's even harder when parents are fighting. The sight or sound of Mom and Dad arguing can traumatize kids.

Whether the divorce is angry or friendly, children are deeply affected. Grief is inevitable, as are the many emotions that accompany it, like anger, fear, and confusion. Questions arise: What will happen now? Who loves me? Will I ever be happy again? A storm of feelings and worries can lead to behaviors that tax already stressed parents. But they are cries for help, unconscious ways children ask for reassurance, love, and understanding.

How you handle the process of separation and divorce will impact how much stress and trauma your child endures. Honest heart-to-heart discussions about what to expect are key to supporting him through this transition, while a strong arsenal of coping skills will help him weather the tensions and challenges of a new family dynamic.[3] This is where the Nine Tools come in. They teach children to find their own stability and navigate the tide of conflicting emotions that might otherwise pull them under. Even if you are years into the process, with regrets behind you, your child's creativity can soothe old hurts and restore his inner peace and happiness. That's what happened with Madison.

Madison's parents hadn't told her they were separating; Dad just quietly moved out. He traveled frequently for business, so they hoped the kids wouldn't notice the change. They couldn't tell them where things were headed because they didn't know themselves. By the time I met Madison, divorce proceedings had begun.

Leaving Mistaken for Not Loving: Madison had a hard time waking up in the morning and facing the day. It was awful to see her parents upset; she wanted them to be happy . . . and back together. She told me her parents must not love her because if they did, they'd stay married.

One Parent Gets the Burden: Madison's behavior worsened around her dad. She refused to talk to him on the phone and didn't want to hear his voice, say his name, or touch his photo. "I don't want to see him," she told me. "I feel like he hates me, like work is more important. And I don't like two homes." But the next day she wrote him, "I love you so much. If you could love me, I could love *me* more."

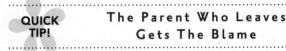

QUICK TIP!

The Parent Who Leaves Gets The Blame

Kids are often angry at the parent who leaves and sorry for the one who stays in the house or resists the separation. They also love both. It's complex and confusing, and adjustment takes time. If you can avoid blaming each other or letting your child see your anger, it will be easier on him.

Parents Apologize: Madison was understandably confused about why her parents had split. They never asked if she had questions or reassured her that it wasn't her fault. Once we started working together, her parents realized how important this was to all the children, and apologized for not telling them earlier. They started having long family discussions—together and apart—and encouraged Madison and her siblings to share whatever was on their minds and in their hearts. This show of respect meant a lot to Madison.

Backup Safe Place for Stress: With her world crumbling, Madison needed sanctuary from stress. I invited her to create a haven. She described "a place where you can survive because the trees have fruit, there are forest animals like foxes, fresh water, and an ocean nearby." In this Special Place, she found quiet respite. "Nothing can attack me," she said. "I'm safe and relaxed."

Animals Offer Support: A nearby lake housed a family of Dolphins. "I can swim and cool off there," she explained, "and if I have no one to talk to, I can talk to them." Her favorite one, Dante, took her "really deep, where I am protected."

Hearts Tear: I had Madison explore how her Heart was faring. She imagined an "ugly brown torn-apart heart." The sides had raw edges with large chunks missing, as if someone had ripped it. One small drop of blue happiness remained on the top left side. I asked her what colors might grow that spot of joy. She looked inside for the answer: "Blow on it with soft blue breath, and water it with cool green rain." She was to do this every morning and night. Breath by breath, and drop by drop, her poor Heart started on a slow path toward healing.

Dreams Foretell the Present: One night Madison dreamed a volcano erupted outside her house. Ten feet away, an earthquake rumbled. She was shocked, scared, and worried about her own safety, yet responsible for rounding up people to go to the basement. When she finally took cover, she fell through a vent. But no one was paying attention. She felt that everyone in the house was running out on her. This was, of course, a thinly disguised metaphor for her disrupted life. "I feel completely out of control," she complained. "And I have to do everything." She drew a storm of random dark colors depicting her feelings about the dream. She titled the picture "Anger and Chaos." That said it all.

Guides to the Rescue: I suggested she call in reinforcements. A Rabbit came and gave her a sword to cut through her fears. An ancient Wizard—111 years old and dressed in a whirling sapphire gown—gave her pink powder to store in her Heart. Whenever she sprinkled it over herself, it would dissolve her worries. "Be wise," Wizard reminded her. "Keep hope, trust, faith, and kindness in your Heart always."

Calmness Triumphs Over Stress: The divorce also took a toll on Madison's body, and she started to experience chest pains. She identified it as *Stress*, a sharp purple pain on the right side of her heart. When I asked if she could locate *Calmness*, she found it on the left side of her heart; it looked like salmon-colored clouds. By breathing Calmness into Stress, she reduced her anxiety from 8 to 1, while Calmness shot up from 2 to 9. Her Heart told her to practice this exercise every night, and three times daily.

More Animal Assistance: One day I asked Madison who or what might open her Heart to new possibilities. A white Tiger appeared. She helped her explore issues she couldn't face on her own, like "feeling okay" about the new living arrangements. Tiger's message was, "Remember to RELAX your body and think of the good things, not the bad. Remember Dad will always be your dad, and Mom will always be your mom." Her Gift was a heart-shaped gold locket engraved with a happy face. Inside it said, "Call me when you need me." These messages took her one step further on her healing journey.

Practicing her new Tools, along with frequent late-night talks with her parents, gave Madison the ability to turn the tide on her sorrow and develop a fresh perspective. She lost

---

EASY HINTS!

Recipe for a "Happy and Good Life"

MADISON'S SECRET FORMULA

Love and Healing
+ Safe Place
+ Animal/Wizard Medicine
+ Positive Thoughts
+ Balloon Breathing
+ Friends
+ Relaxation Tapes
− Yelling
= Happiness!

weight, made peace with her siblings, and began to enjoy life again—in two homes. Within months, her healing Heart finally smiled. It was happy true blue with a big green grin. Madison developed her own self-success formula (page 186), gleaned from all our work together and her own recovering joy. She hoped it could make a difference for other kids going through their parents' split.

HOW-TO FOR YOU

Whether you are thinking about separation, in the middle of divorce, or dealing with the aftermath, your child can use his imagination to heal his Heart and face the future. Although it's best to have quiet time set aside for this work, it's not always possible. Don't let that stop you. Many of these tasks and topics can be incorporated into everyday conversation. As always, work with what you have.

⚎ Speak the Truth

Discuss the situation calmly and clearly. It's great if parents can do this together. If not, take the reins yourself. Let him know that this is not his fault and that he will be taken care of. He may need lots of reassurance and ask the same questions repeatedly: "Where will I live? When will I see each of you?" Be patient and answer as best you can. Remind him that Mom and Dad love him and will always be his parents. No one is divorcing *him*.

⚎ Make Feelings Visible

Separation and divorce stir up big feelings in kids: hurt, sadness, betrayal, fear. They may show up as poor behavior, but the real culprits are feelings, not actions. Encourage your child to voice and accept his emotions. Have him draw them or talk to them directly. Where do they live in his body? What do they look like? What do they need to express right now? What do they need to feel better?

Cure with Color

Have your child explore his feelings through color. What colors are his *Hurt* feelings? His *Fear*? His *Sadness*? What colors might make those better? See how breathing in different colors can move him from Fear to *Trust*, from Hurt to *Hopeful*.

Team Up to Care for Tender Hearts

Animal Friends and Wizards make great mentors during the pain of parental divorce. They offer your child the wealth of his own deep resources and resilience. Support him going to his inner safe place and calling upon creative helpers. He can say, "I hate that my parents don't love each other anymore. How can I stop hurting? What can I do so I don't feel stuck in the middle?" These guides often know what he needs.

Rely on Dreams

Dreams are one way that children process turmoil. They offer information from deep levels of the subconscious. Invite your child to share his dreams each morning through talking, drawing, or writing—it will motivate him to remember them. Like fables, they provide meanings or lessons. Have fun using intuition to figure them out. No need to analyze every detail; just sharing is cathartic.

Create a Safety Zone

Children internalize everything. They love you both, and your anger splits their loyalties. Create battle-free zones in their presence. Don't fight or criticize each other in front of them. And promote a good relationship with your ex. Your kids need to love you both without guilt or confusion.

Tolerate the Hoping Heart

Almost all children of divorce hope their parents will reunite. Even years later. Sometimes even after parents remarry. Be clear and patient when explaining what will or will not happen, but understand that this fantasy is normal.

- **Bandage Old Wounds**
  What if the divorce and the damage are already done? It's not too late. Ask your child what he would have liked to be different. Talk directly to his Heart and ask what it needs to forgive and heal. It may be something you can do, or he may need to call in a special guide.

When Fido or Kitty Dies

How to Cope With the Loss of a Pet

Will had known Smoke all his life—seven whole years! The black Lab slept at the foot of his bed and greeted him, tail wagging, whenever he got home. He happily let Will dress him in cowboy hats and bandanas. When Smoke died, Will was grief-stricken. Inconsolable, he refused to eat or play with his buddies, and he suffered from stomachaches and crying jags.

The loss of a pet is often a child's first experience with death, and it can be devastating. Pets are trusted companions who offer unconditional love, and losing one can leave a hole in a child's heart. It can also raise questions about the nature of living and dying, which is a difficult concept for young minds to handle. A child's imagination, however, will help him unravel his beliefs and feelings, reduce his anxiety, and create a healing connection with his beloved creature. Will's certainly did.

Nauseous—Just Like the Dog: Will came to me struggling with nausea and a fear of "throw-up." Smoke had been visibly ill at the end of his life, and Will's despair was making him equally sick. He worried about vomiting and got frightened if anyone else did. He imagined the vomit color throughout his body, and it freaked him out. We needed to deal with this right away.

Animal Tums for the Tummy: After a few calming Balloon Breaths, Will called in an Animal Friend for assistance. A frightened Deer, just learning to be brave, showed up. He advised Will to walk away if he saw anyone throw up at school, or go play with his friends and forget about it. Deer gave Will the Gift of a *Courage Stone* to enable him to breathe slowly and leave the scene. When he did, everything would smell good again. And as Will's courage grew, so did Deer's, as he turned into the majestic being he truly was.

QUICK TIP! Animals Are Often Mirrors

Not every Animal Friend who shows up will be brave or wise. A scared child might picture a skittish Rabbit or a nervous Deer. That's okay. Kids often reach for guides who understand them right where they are. Welcome each Animal Friend and listen to its counsel. Your child's imagination may be wiser than both of you.

Doggie Heaven Brings Comfort: Will's nausea seemed to do double duty—it distracted him from his deep feelings and kept him close to Smoke, but not in a healing way. I asked Will, "What happens when someone dies?" He said they went to Heaven, and he told me Smoke was in Doggie Heaven, a happy place above the clouds where cats were forbidden. Dogs there could climb on furniture, eat anything they wanted, and scratch themselves with a special pole. Smoke played with departed canine friends and family, like his littermates and a neighbor's terrier. "People whose dogs die can visit," he explained. I asked him to draw a picture of Doggie Heaven to remind himself that Smoke was somewhere good and happy.

Memories Lift Spirits: We also explored Will's favorite memories: walking with Smoke and Dad in the rain, playing dress-up, taking family pictures, Smoke licking his face in the morning or playing alone together . . . all the way back to when Will was a baby. Telling stories, with the laughter and tears they evoked, was a comforting and cathartic way to process his grief. As he did so, Will's nausea evaporated.

Visit from Above: Of course, Will missed Smoke terribly. Nothing would change that. But I wondered what would happen if Will imagined him coming to visit. He could do that easily and envisioned Smoke floating down from Doggie Heaven on blue angel wings. He arrived with a Frisbee in his teeth, ready to play like a puppy. They jumped and laughed on the front lawn. This connection with Smoke's spirit eased some of Will's loneliness.

Heartache Lessens Over Time: Six weeks later, Will took a close look at his Heart. He drew two pictures of it. The first, his past, was distraught; its eyes were shut with heavy tears, and it wore a fierce frown. His present Heart was healing. The tears lingered, but they were lighter, and his sadness lessened. At twelve weeks, it lifted more. On a scale of 0 to 10, his Heart went from sadness 9 and happiness 2 to sadness 3 and happiness 8. He was almost his normal joyful self.

QUICK TIP!   Time Heals Wounds

We can't put a time limit on grief. Depending on the severity of the loss, it can last days, weeks, months, or years. It might take less time to grieve over a new goldfish than a favorite cat or dog. But it might not. Let your child go through her process at her own pace.

Will took the time he needed to deal with his grief and frolicked with a new puppy the following year.

HOW-TO FOR YOU

Will's love for Smoke endured, yet his Heart healed. These ideas can help your child as well.

▓ Ask What Happens When Someone Dies

Your child's beliefs about death often reflect your family views, even if you haven't discussed them directly. And children pick up and make up all kinds of ideas about death and dying, some of which frighten them and others that bring comfort. Use this time to begin talking about the cycle of life. Allow your child to have her own comforting vision right now. Have her draw or describe what she imagines.

▓ Create Space and Time for Grief

You might want to run out and find another pet right away, thinking it will ease the suffering. Wait. Respect her sadness and give her time to mourn fully.

▓ Counting Down Sorrow

Check in regularly with your child's Heart; use the 0 to 10 Scale to gauge where she is in the grief process. If her sorrow is intense or her good feelings are low, you know she's still in the early stages, and there is more healing to do. Continue to use the Tools to release her grief and nourish her happiness. Eventually the numbers will change.

▓ Say a Final Good-bye

If your child didn't get to say a real good-bye to her pet, she can always imagine one. What would she say if he were here now? How might he reply? They can "talk" this way whenever she likes.

❖ Visit Animal Heaven

Many children believe that their dog or cat goes on to a Special Place for pets, like Will's Doggie Heaven. If your child is one of these, she can go there using her Heart's imagination. Use the Special Place script to help her find her way, then ask, "What's it like there? How different is it from here? What do they do all day?" This ability to "visit" her four-footed friend will surely soothe. And perhaps puppy or kitty spirits can return the visit. They can play together as her Heart tugs.

❖ Great Animals Don't Leave

The same Tools that let your child connect with imagined Animal Friends can maintain a connection to her real, but departed, pet. Invisible ribbons can represent the love connecting their Hearts. Telling stories also keeps good memories alive. Some kids imagine their pets as Animal Friend guides who watch over them. As time passes, ask if that's a possibility. It can be a great comfort.

When the Most Horrible Happens

How to Manage When a Loved One Dies

Heather was the sweetest nine-year-old. She was cooperative and kind, a delight to her family, friends, and teachers. So when her dad died of cancer, Heather put on a brave front; she didn't complain or cry in public. But she started pulling out her eyebrows—one tiny blond hair at a time—until they were all gone, mimicking her dad's hair loss during chemotherapy. That's when her worried mom brought her to me.

Death is always difficult for children to grasp. And when a family member dies, it's even harder. All the usual emotional and behavioral turmoil of loss come out in force. There may also be reactions specific to this kind of significant loss. For instance, young kids don't comprehend the permanency of death; they may repeat the same questions: "Where is Nana? When is she coming back? Is she still dead?" When they do understand, it can raise more frightened questions: "Will you die? Will I die? What will happen?" They may also generalize cause and effect: If Grandpa died in his sleep, they may fear bedtime.

Some children take on attributes of their loved one to keep him alive; others direct their pain inward, neglecting or harming themselves. Conflicting emotions are common. A bereaved child might sob uncontrollably one moment, then play with his friends as if nothing happened the next. Children grieve in spurts; intense emotions are hard to handle for too long. Once grief seems to have passed, it can make periodic comebacks. Holidays, birthdays, school events, and family gatherings are common triggers.

No one "gets over" a significant loss like the death of a parent or sibling, but kids are resilient and can learn to live with a new reality. They need to feel important, involved, and safe enough to go through the mourning process. They need a place where they can experience loss and still feel nurtured. The goal is to transform the relationship with their departed loved one from a day-to-day presence into one of healthy and supportive memories. That's what I hoped to offer Heather; her imagination was the way to get there.

When I first met Heather, she didn't seem to be actively grieving. But sorrow was just below the surface, waiting for the right moment to emerge.

Anger Makes an Appearance: I met her anger first. It was "like a black storm," she said, filling the entire top of her head. First she lost her dad, and now her mom was selling the house. It was more change than she could bear. She was angry about all of it—everything that wasn't like it used to be. "If Dad didn't die, we wouldn't have to do this," she complained. "All Mom does is talk about Dad; she doesn't seem to care about me."

Black and Red Bring Catharsis: Heather's anger was so strong that I had her draw it. She scribbled feverishly with black and red markers. After fifteen minutes, there was hardly a white spot left on the paper, and it was shredded in places. When she had finished, she collapsed, sobbing.

Anger Hides Sorrow: Heather was afraid she'd never stop crying. Her anger covered an aching heart. She missed her dad so much. She believed he was in Heaven, and the idea of connecting to him was the only thing that soothed her. I suggested she imagine her dad sending love from above. Deep pink love flowed to her from Dad's spirit hands, turning her sad gray Heart pink. As Dad's love reached Heather, her sorrow momentarily subsided, and her Heart returned to its natural loving state. She pictured little pink hearts coming down from Heaven and filling her body until no empty space was left.

Hearts Rule: Heather painted fuchsia hearts scattered across the largest ocean she could imagine, an expression of how much she loved her father. And she drew a self-portrait holding a smiling teddy bear in a T-shirt, close to her own Heart. I asked her to consider the possibility of taking better care of herself and leaving her eyebrows alone.

The Great Divide: We turned to Heart and Belly for further insight. Heather's Heart was trying to help her be kinder to herself and accept her current life. But her Belly feelings didn't want to listen. Belly was still upset and wanted Heather to pull out eyebrows and "maybe my eyelashes." He didn't want to change, but was distressed by the way she treated herself. "He doesn't like when I pick my eyebrows because it hurts me," she explained "But he's mad at Heart, although she's right."

Backtrack Alert

Imageries may produce mixed messages. Feelings can change drastically from moment to moment, or Body Parts can hold conflicting opinions. That's okay. A child may want to change—mostly—but part of him might not, or he doesn't know how. Even adults hold opposing truths at the same time. It's natural. The process may feel like a roller coaster, but go along for the ride. As long as your child expresses his feelings, healing is happening.

Stomach and Heart Compromise: Heather needed a win-win solution to resolve this power struggle. I asked if Belly would be willing to compromise with Heart. Belly said yes and confessed his fear that Heart was taking over. Heart explained that she just wanted to show Heather a more healing path. They agreed to tell her—together—to "stop hurting and being mean" to herself. Heather agreed to try.

Use What You Have: One week Heather arrived wearing a lovely Native American necklace. It had five totem birds strung between turquoise beads—a gift from her dad's sister. It was her "good luck necklace," she recounted, and the birds were like the five members of her family, Dad included. These little "animal angels" turned out to be perfect helpers. Heather closed her eyes and imagined herself walking along a healing path. She found a cozy place to rest and, one by one, touched each bird. In her fantasy, they took flight and shared their wisdom and Gifts.

Animal Angels Bring Gifts: The jade Canary gave her the Gift of *Knowledge* to make good choices about her eyebrows. The opal Eagle carried a *Heart Box* in his beak. Whenever Heather placed her hopes inside, Eagle would fly them to her dad in Heaven. The pink quartz Parrot gave her a *Rose* to track her progress. As Heather's eyebrows grew back, the flower grew, too. "This bird teaches me that if I make smart choices, I will have a big flower," she explained. Brown Sparrow gave her the Gift of *Kindness* so she could treat herself with respect. The final friend was a turquoise Hummingbird that crooned, "Be normal, not perfect." This angel gave Heather a *Trumpet* to call anyone in the world to be with her. As she held the necklace in her hands, the birds sang in chorus: "Use the Gifts wisely."

QUICK TIP!   It's Always Improv

Imagery always involves improvisation; that's why the same Tools work in radically different situations. Watch for unexpected prompts—like Heather's new necklace—and see what ideas they suggest. The Nine Tools are just one part of your child's healing journey. Your own imagination and insight are the other.

Heart and Belly Become Faithful Friends: As Heather's healing journey continued, I invited her to reconnect with Heart and Belly wisdom. Her Heart was still "clear and pink"; so was its message: "Do what keeps you calm. Listen inside. Stay focused on not picking eyebrows." Belly agreed and reminded her to always listen to Heart, "because she is wise."

Check-ups Required: A few weeks later, we checked in with Heart again. She was proud because Heather's eyebrows were growing. I asked Heather if there was any part of her that still wanted to pluck. She closed her eyes, connected to her inner voice, and noticed that her hands still had the urge. "They know I have a lot of stress about Dad, and pulling lets go of it." Her hands didn't care how Heart felt; they wanted to release their own tension. Stress was "gray like a cloud" that lived in her hands and brain. When I asked her to find an antistress color, "solid pink and white" appeared immediately.

Breathe in Antistress: I suggested she breathe in her antistress colors. As she did, the gray cloud in her hands left through her fingers, and the one in her brain, through her ears. With them went the urge to pull; only one percent was left. Heather continued this exercise at home whenever she needed it.

The Value of Understanding: Eventually Heather was strong enough to wonder how this hair pulling had begun. She checked inside and acknowledged how miserable she'd been when her father died; she'd needed something to do with her pain. Pulling a tiny eyebrow hair had seemed harmless. "I was really upset and didn't know how to control the urge," she confessed. I wondered if she was ready to find a way to bring joy and happiness into her life. She was, but wasn't sure how. I suggested a Wizard might be right for the task.

Wizard Brings Joy: A young, happy Wizard appeared. He let her know that if she allowed *Joy* in, it would reduce her sad thinking. He gave her a turquoise velvet bag that contained a book and a bubble maker. The book was called *How to Bring Joy and Happiness into My Life.* Anytime she opened it, she would find an easy "happiness starting" suggestion. The bubble maker came with instructions to blow bubbles whenever she felt like tugging at her eyebrows. The bubbles would catch the desire and carry it away.

> ### EASY HINTS!
>
> **What I can do for myself . . .**
>
> #### HEATHER'S HEART SPEAKS
>
> 1 Practice the Balloon Breath.
> 2 Relax my muscles and my bones.
> 3 Surround myself with good light and happiness.
> 4 Find my Special Place.
> 5 Listen to my Heart.
> 6 Get my anger out.
> 7 Listen to my Animal Angels.
> 8 Try not to be perfect.

As Heather used her imagination to move through her grief, she began to take better care of herself. Her eyebrows and her happiness grew in beautifully. She still missed her dad every day, but she learned to appreciate her life. At night she dreamed of flying in a love-propelled spaceship to visit her dad in Heaven. And she knew he would always be close at Heart.

Above are some of her favorite practices for taking good care of herself.

HOW-TO FOR YOU

Heather used her Heart and her imagination to face the intense grief of her father's death. The same Tools may enable your child to deal with loss.

Set Aside Time to Share

Many kids bottle up big feelings, but sorrow doesn't need to be contained. Set up a time when tears and fears can flow. Listen to his Heart's woes without fixing them. Just acknowledge that you hear him and that his emotions are valid.

Give Reassurance

Answer your child's questions simply and honestly. He won't ask for more information than he can handle, so let his questions guide you. Reassure him that he is safe and you will be there for him.

Create a Safe Haven

Encourage your child to imagine a Special Place—a private sanctuary where he can escape the painful changes in his life. Have him surround himself with anything or anyone that might help him heal.

Offer a Bowl of Hearts

Hearts can hurt, and hearts can comfort. Have your child check in with his, to see what soothing words or pictures he discovers. Write his Heart's messages on cards and keep them in a bowl. If need be, offer a few choices like, "Be gentle with yourself. You have a big heart. You are on the right road. Allow yourself time to heal. It's okay to enjoy good things in life." He can pull one whenever sweet words are needed.

Connect with Loved Ones

Spend family time looking at pictures and sharing memories. Your child may want to keep mementos by his bed—a piece of clothing, jewelry, or a photo. It's important for him to understand that just because people are absent doesn't mean they've left his heart or his life.

Wise Guides Bring Gifts

Animal Friends and Wizards can be a comforting presence. Their messages and Gifts often respond to his secret yearnings and offer a wisdom no one else can provide. Some children imagine their missing loved one as a visitor or guardian angel. It's another way to adjust and feel connected in this new reality.

Remember, Grief Is a Process

Be patient. Your child will move through this loss at the pace his heart can handle.

Grief Comfort
Imagery for a Hurting Heart

This gentle meditation will help your child use his inner resources to move through his grief and repair his hurting heart. Before bed is a natural time to take this journey, as well as anytime during the day that emotions are running high.

Let's take some time to be gentle with you. You deserve lots of extra care right now. Allow your eyes to softly close and slow your breathing. Pay attention to your breath as you imagine walking down a path to find your safe Special Place. As you enter through the door, this time things might be a little bit different. Your safe place is set up to fit your special needs. It has become a Room of Comfort. Notice what it looks like. How it is designed just for you. You may find soft, warm pillows and objects or toys you love.

Consider your Heart. What does it feel like now? What picture does it present? What does it need? Surround yourself with those who love you. They could be people or animals . . . alive or departed. Notice who shows up. What do they look like? Are they different from what you thought? They are here to support you and ease any suffering.

Share your troubles with them. It's safe to let your Heart speak. It's okay to cry. It's okay to laugh. All your feelings are fine. You may feel sadness and loss. You may be scared. You may be angry about what happened. You might worry about the future. Or feel guilty about something you said or did. Know that nothing you did or said caused this loss. You may also feel nothing at all. Anything you feel—or don't feel—is fine.

Notice if your emotions have colors . . . shapes . . . or pictures. Perhaps some have messages for you. They may speak to you or give you a Gift to help you handle your unhappiness.

So might your people and Animal Friends. They are all wise and loving.

They have so much to explain about what you are going through. Maybe they all want to speak at once. If so, ask them to take turns. Let each one come close—one by one—and share his or her important message for letting your Heart heal.

And they might not speak, but may hold you close and keep you safe. You can collapse in their arms or hide at their side. Whatever you need, whatever feels right, your friends and family are there for you. Tell them. They want to help.

It's also okay to take time out from your grieving. To forget about your troubles and play or run or read or laugh or do anything that takes your mind away. Let yourself take a break from your heavy Heart.

Love and support are all around you as you go through this pain. Allow your friends' and family's love to sink into your being, your body, your heart. Ask for help whenever you want. Take all the time you need to have this experience. You can return to this Comfort Room anytime you want. When you're ready, be aware of your breathing, your body, and return here, keeping all you have learned in your Heart.

CHAPTER 10

When Good Kids Do Bad
Things . . . To Themselves
and Others

Helping Your Child Handle Anger,
Hurt, and Frustration

**My brain and my heart
are stronger than my mad
feelings.**
—*Danny, age seven*

N o one is perfect. Yet we often demand it of others and ourselves. So we set expectations too high, become disappointed or frustrated, and then get angry, often making choices we regret. "We're only human," we say. "Everyone gets angry." And it's true. Everyone does get angry. It's a healthy survival mechanism that tells us our welfare is threatened and something is wrong or needs changing. And because our sense of well-being extends beyond physical safety, unacknowledged feelings of disappointment, anxiety, and hurt can also ignite anger. Children are no different, except they have less practice expressing their feelings and less developed reasoning centers, making anger a common quick-fix solution.

There is, however, a difference between angry feelings and angry behavior or aggression. Anger is normal and inevitable, but aggressive behavior can be hurtful, disruptive, and self-destructive. In fact, unchecked aggression can create family turmoil, problems at school, broken friendships, and physical and emotional harm. Lashing out, crying, and yelling are common fallback positions when a child's tender feelings are bruised. Frustration, embarrassment, loneliness and isolation, even difficult transitions may lead to bursts of fury. While blame—anger's sly cousin—may try to absolve the irate child of responsibility for any of it.[1]

Ten-year-old Meredith's anger was triggered by simple decisions. She got so frustrated choosing what to wear or what movie to see that she'd stamp her feet and run out of the room, slamming doors behind her. Seven-year-old Jon hurt his playmates' feelings with spiteful barbs but sobbed that they all hated him whenever they complained. And one little girl was so worn down by her big sister's taunts that she confessed to her mother, "I want to kill her."

Rage is explosive in a small body; the heart pounds and muscles tense, and that energy seeks release. It's a hot-wired response, the primitive part of the brain (the *amygdala*) discharging enough adrenaline to fight or run away from an enemy. It is only our "modern" brain, the *frontal lobe*, which allows us to respond to anger signals with reason and problem solving.[2] But children don't have well-developed frontal lobes; their brains and reason are still growing, fed by experience and the assimilation of newly learned coping skills. While these increase a child's self-control and help him bounce back from stress, they also contribute to better health, social relationships, and academic performance. Therefore it's important that children learn effective and healthy ways of controlling their anger.[3]

Most kids do. It's a routine part of growing up. Around preschool, kids learn to "use their words" to express feelings instead of yelling, pushing, pinching, or biting. As they grow, they acquire more sophisticated language skills and develop empathy. Understanding the effect their words and actions have on others helps children learn to cooperate and compromise. By late elementary school, they are typically able to express their anger verbally instead of physically and are ready to consider anger as a problem to be solved.[4]

Some children, however, require more direct guidance and practice. Perhaps they never had the chance or need to learn these skills. Perhaps a new life crisis—a move, the birth of a baby sister, or change of school—has thrown their systems off and they are regressing. A very young child may simply be in the first throes of learning anger management skills; each outburst then becomes a new teaching opportunity.

Imagination is the perfect tutor. The Nine Tools can teach children to control and reduce bad tempers. It gives them access to the emotions behind their anger and teaches them to calm themselves and gain perspective. Scarlet, eleven, was a walking fury; when she drew a self-portrait, red *Anger* filled her entire body. But when she imagined *Love* as a soft shower washing over her, her anger began to subside. Tyrone, nine, was a bully at school until he learned to breathe in pale blue *Calmness* and white *Love*, which scattered his explosive feelings; he changed his reputation and made new friends. As one sixth-grade boy put it, "I like imagery because it helps me slow down and cool off. I can think about relaxing and not be so mean."

This chapter examines the hurts, angers, and frustrations that make kids act out in both small and harmful ways. You'll learn to help your child manage those times when he's filled with hurt or rage and teach him to access these skills on his own.

When Little Ones Can't Manage

How to Channel Frustration and Other Anger Neighbors

Almost six, Erica was soft-spoken and sensitive. She played the piano, cared for the family pets, and was generally kind and gentle . . . except when she wasn't. Then she would become rude and stubborn, refusing to take "no" for an answer. She would yell, cry, argue, hit, and regularly drive everyone crazy. What no one saw was the frustration under all that noise. As the youngest of four, Erica found it hard to get the attention she needed from her busy parents. Bigger voices always seemed to draw their notice. "No one listens when I'm talking," she complained. And while her parents understood how she felt, they often played it down. After all, in such a chaotic household, everyone felt a little short-changed.

But Erica was too young to understand. And since she had not yet learned appropriate ways to get love and attention, she pulled focus any way she could. Screaming worked well. Hitting was equally effective. Everyone noticed her then. And her distraught parents watched their sweet, gentle girl turn into a fuming terror.

Erica's demanding behavior spilled over to school. She started pushing and scratching her friends when they wouldn't play with her. Her teacher requested a "shadow" aid so she didn't hurt her classmates. Mom and Dad tried to handle her behavior themselves, but when Erica "pulled a fork" on her sister at breakfast, they finally sought outside help.

Whenever I see anger, I look for the feelings behind it. Children experience big emotions—big fear, big frustration, big hurt—and they don't always know how to express them in ways adults can hear. They may find their emotions frightening and deny them, although their behavior tells a different story. Very young children may not yet have language for their emotions. Their big feelings are like enormous waves that catch them in the undertow. Bad behavior is their desperate attempt to stay afloat. But once a child can quiet his anger, he can explore where it comes from. And by addressing his core emotions, we can disarm his aggression and teach him new skills. That was my plan for Erica.

When I met Erica, she felt enormous guilt about her behavior. Her sense of self was shattered, and all she could say was, "I am a bad girl."

Simplify with a Graph: "Good" and "bad" are among the first distinctions a small child makes. They were the only words Erica initially had to explain her complex feelings, and bad was Big. She described it as "black, black, black." To get a clearer picture, I made a simple graph: a long thin rectangle with the number 10 at the top, a zero (0) at the bottom, and a 5 in the middle. "The top," I explained, "is the most bad you can feel; the bottom is not feeling bad at all." I asked Erica how she felt, and she pointed near the top. We did the same for her good feelings; they were at the bottom. When she realized there weren't many good feelings, she wanted more. So we made it a goal for the following week: "More good feelings!"

Black and Gold—Together and Apart: Erica felt better after she left my office. Talking about what happened and how she felt about her behavior, without being judged, lifted her spirits and gave her hope. But without skills to sustain her, she quickly reverted to her angry routine. She came back keen to do better and try something new. I asked her to imagine where the bad black part lived inside her. "Everywhere," she said. I wondered if there was any good in there at all, and she admitted to a tiny gold speck in her Heart. She wanted to feel more of it but couldn't imagine how. I suggested she breathe in that speck of good gold into the bad black part and see what happened. To her amazement, bad started to turn good.

Illustrate What's Going On: I invited Erica to draw two pictures: how she felt when she arrived and how she was feeling now. The results were striking: In the first, she drew herself with a big frown and no arms; tears marked her face. In her "after" picture, she had a big smile, feet firmly planted, and large hands that might (I hoped) reach out to others.

Red Hearts Deliver: Now that we had diffused her dark feelings, it was time to give Erica take-home skills. I taught her the Balloon

Breath and, because she was so young, gave her a red glass heart to hold when she practiced. This enchanted her, and her parents made a small pouch so she could carry it around her neck. Holding this tiny object gave her something *to do* while focusing on her breathing; it served as an anchor and a reminder of what she had learned.

Advice of the Panda: We then turned to animals to look for inner wisdom. I asked Erica about her favorite creatures. After her own dog and cat, she loved panda bears. Since little kids sometimes need a gentle kick-start for imagination work, I took the lead and assigned Panda as her special Animal Friend. I asked her to close her eyes and imagine Panda whispering something helpful to her; perhaps offering her a Gift. She heard him right away. He said, "Be kind" and gave her the Gift of a *Caring Heart*. Not surprising, since I had given her that small heart the week before.

QUICK TIP!   **You Add Your Own Magic**

Children take to heart everything you say and give them. As a result, your observations, suggestions, and gifts have extra power; they may even show up days later as part of their imagination wisdom.

Red Bull Protects: To bring little Erica to another level of understanding, I wondered aloud if these big bad feelings were mad, or sad, or scared. Having a choice helped her realize they were *Mad* feelings. She seemed ready to deal with them, so I suggested she imagine where Mad lived and what it looked like. She closed her eyes and envisioned a Red Bull in her right knee. She explained he was there to protect her from the Red Bull in other people. I had her ask what might calm him down; did any images, thoughts, or words come to mind? She pictured a white filter, stored in her ankle, which could be expanded to fit her throat to change her angry tone. That way, when the Bull came out, he still defended Erica, but wasn't "so mean."

Pink Potion Dissolves Anger: Was there anything else she needed to be aware of? Erica conjured a potion of pink *Love*. It was kept in her Heart and could calm her Bull. Whenever he drank the love brew, it put him to sleep, his sharp horns rounded, and he got "happier, smaller, and turned a calm blue." This concoction was more powerful than the white filter, which was now relegated to backup, "If I don't get the potion in time."

Energy Does the Trick: When Erica mentioned Panda's Gift of a *Heart*, I realized my gift had touched her. Her own vulnerable Heart would be a good place to continue the work. We played an energy game. I put my hand on her back, just behind her Heart center, and had her guess what color I was pulling out and what color was going in. She said I was pulling out gray and black and putting in pink and red. These colors matched her bad/mad and love feelings. "So I don't hurt anyone, and I can be nice," she volunteered. I then had her do something similar for herself. As she touched her own Heart, she breathed in Love and breathed out Anger, letting it simply melt away. She was learning to calm herself. Now she needed to express herself in more appropriate ways. We called for extra Animal assistance.

A Giraffe Named Bartholomew: Erica expected Panda to reappear. But a huge Giraffe showed up. His name was Bartholomew, and he understood Erica's predicament. Because he was so tall, and his head was in the trees, other animals often forgot he was there. When he wanted their attention, he didn't get mad. He just gently lowered his head, looked them in the eye, and softly said what he wanted. Most of the time, they listened. But if they were busy, he found something fun to do, like eating leaves, and tried again later. Erica laughed and decided to try this approach at home, except for the eating leaves part. Maybe she could play by herself for a while, too.

Sasha, the Self-Control Wizard: For final assistance, we called in the big guns: Wizard Wisdom. A stunning Self-Control Wizard was waiting in the wings. I encouraged Erica to talk with her alone. "I feel her in my Heart," she reported back. "Sasha gives me pretty notes like 'Always let your heart shine.' and 'I'll teach you to be a good friend even when you aren't in the mood.' And she says she'll show up whenever I need her."

Erica was delighted by her imagination skills and relished the praise for her new cooperative behavior. The family also made changes. Mom started taking her to lunch for special alone time. Dad initiated Sunday Kid Outings: Each week a different child had him for the entire morning. And Erica returned to being the sweet, gentle girl that everyone remembered.

HOW-TO FOR YOU

Erica started out expressing her anger destructively, but with the Tools of her imagination, she learned how to be a happier child. Your child can, too.

❖ Make Simple Graphs

Help your child face his angry feelings with a graph or pie chart. A bar graph is easier for a little kid to understand. Have him imagine how much anger (or hurt or frustration) he's feeling; then ask how much he'd like to feel. Make that his goal. As he applies the Nine Tools, check in for weekly progress.

An older child might prefer a pie chart. How much of

his emotional life is anger? What percentage is loving or peaceful? Would he like to slice his life pie differently? Use whatever Tools that appeal to him to get there.

Examine Rage Gently

It's not easy for a child to admit how angry he is, so jokes about being a Grumpy Grouch or Angry Ant can backfire. A gentle approach will soften his defenses. Try wondering what his different feelings look like, where he feels them in his body, or what cartoon characters they remind him of. He can then sketch or paint his creations.

This can be a door opener to talking more directly about his anger—or what's really bothering him. Ask him one or two questions like, "I'd like to understand what are you angry about. What are your thoughts about what made you so mad? How would you like things to be different?" However, go slow and don't push. This is a tender conversation and can't be rushed. See what he's open to, and use your judgment.

Play with Puppets

With very young kids, even a drawing might feel abstract. Paper bag puppets are great for working out conflicting feelings. Just two paper bags and some crayons and, *voilà*, you have angry/calm stand-ins who, with your child's assistance, can actually talk to each other and work it out.

Find a Token for Comfort

Pick an object from a fun vacation—a stone, a shell, a small toy, whatever strikes his fancy. Have your child hold it and picture that special time—with all its sounds, smells, and colors—whenever his steam starts to rise. It can distract him and diffuse the moment. Once calm is restored, he can use Imagination Tools to solve the problem. It's good to rehearse in calm times so the "magic" object can take him to that special time when he's in a crisis.

Use Inside Help

The images or characters your child creates for anger can hold the key to his solutions. For instance, if Firestone Fury shows up, ice-cold stones might cool him. Disappointed Daisy can be watered with the magic rain of possibility. Like Animal Friends and Wizards, these personal creations can offer advice or antidotes—all your child has to do is listen.

Take Advantage of Loving Energy

Suggest your child imagine letting go of his anger by visualizing love pouring in. Assist with your loving hands and hugs. Picture pulling out the bad and replacing it with good. Play a game with colors like I did with Erica.

When Big Ones Have Bad Habits

How to Tame an Over-the-Top Temper

Ten-year-old Brody was never at a loss for words. From early on, he told his parents exactly what he thought and felt. But sometimes, talking wasn't enough. He would throw and punch whatever was close by—books, furniture, or a wall, as if he'd never left the terrible twos. His parents knew Brody had problems handling disappointment, but his rages were worsening. He fought over the smallest things: what was for breakfast, where to sit in the car, whose fault it was if a book fell from his backpack. Playdates turned awful. If a pal canceled, Brody would cry and call him a liar. Then he'd turn on his younger sister, yelling or pushing her. "I don't care!" he would shout when his dad tried to intervene.

His parents tried everything—from time-outs to warm, calming baths, from lectures to quiet attempts at reason. Nothing worked. If they got mad at him, Brody sulked in guilt or escalated his anger. Sent to his room, he would bang doors or threaten to jump out the window. These rants scared his sister so much she hid under her bed. Once the outburst was over, Brody was fine... except the damage was done. His exhausted parents saw him as a walking time bomb and tiptoed around him.

Where does such fury come from? Brody's parents were mellow people who rarely argued. There was nothing in their home that indicated trauma. He did have a penchant for angry rap music, but was that enough to cause such rage? It's not always apparent where anger comes from. Feelings are not linear. Some kids seem to arrive with a bad temper; others may be super-sensitive to the pressures and negative messages around them and react accordingly. Brody had both. And while girls are more likely than boys to have trouble expressing angry feelings, the challenge for some boys is to convey their impulses in words, not deeds.[5]

Imagery Tools can be the mind's own sedative. A child's imagination can teach her to relax in chaos—even chaos of her own making—and free her up to make alternate, more positive choices. It was time for Brody to be his own bomb squad and restore peace to his life.

Locate Anger... and Other Feelings: Brody had so much emotion bubbling up inside that he didn't know what to do with it all. To help him get a handle on it, I had him focus on his Balloon Breath, and one by one, locate where in his body he held different feelings. Then he drew them. There was a lot more than anger going on.

Feelings Show Up in Multiples: White *Worry* arose in his elbow, shoulder, and stomach. Black *Frustration* was under his chin and in his back, where it created a huge hole. Purple *Hurt* lived in his temples, ears, and arms. *Disappointment* was gray and turned up as a huge block in his neck. *Anger* was a combination of all four; it seeped into his internal organs and affected his feet. Brody drew a picture of a broken-down, dejected boy; hardly anything was left of him.

QUICK TIP!   **Anger Comes Second**

Anger surfaces so fast that it steals the limelight; it's easy to miss the deeper feelings underneath. But look past anger, and you often find the real players: sadness, hurt, disappointment, frustration, or betrayal. These are fragile feelings, and anger often runs out first to protect them.

Focus on the Positive: We then looked for positive emotions that Brody could use to create balance. Blue *Calm* was in the top of his head, in his chest, and above his ankles. *Brave* brown was in his thighs and knees, while *Happiness* was a sunny yellow splash in his trunk and hands. Red *Love* was in his heart and toes. When we realized that *Anger* (in his foot) was sandwiched between the Calm in his ankles and the Love in his toes, we had a plan.

Play with Positive Possibilities: Brody breathed in Calm blue, which melted Anger and washed away Worry. Happiness diffused Disappointment, pushing it out into the ground to disintegrate. And Love transformed Frustration and Hurt. In fact, Love seemed to be an all-purpose healer. "When Love moves up my body, it vanishes my bad feelings," Brody noted.

Listen to Heart and Belly Messages: Love in Brody's Heart told him to stay calm and try to do his best. Belly, filled with Bravery and Happiness, suggested he practice Balloon Breathing and remember to be as kind as he could. Belly thought Brody was in pretty bad shape; he wanted him to practice fifteen minutes every hour, but Brody negotiated a more reasonable schedule: three times a day, for one minute each, even on his busiest days. He also promised to shoot hoops in the backyard if the breathing wasn't enough. He was pleased with what he accomplished and resolved to go home and teach his family what he learned.

Anger Payback: Brody sincerely wanted to control himself, but he was still learning these skills and often faltered, displacing his frustration on family and friends. In the process, he unwittingly hurt himself as well. His intense anger often emerged as stomachaches, headaches, and muscle spasms. One day he arrived in my office, body aching from an angry weekend.

Throat Has Something to Say: Brody's neck and throat seemed to be completely locked up. No wonder he was having trouble expressing himself. We used the Three-Question Exercise (page 117) to relieve the physical pain. As Brody looked inward, he got a clear picture of the weight, color, and intensity of his discomfort. *Pain* was a "black blobby knot" that took up a large section of his neck. It started out at a whopping 200 pounds, but as he breathed slowly between rounds of questions, his body relaxed and Pain transformed. Almost immediately, it dropped to 100 pounds and went from black to gray. By the third set of visualizations, it had reduced another 50 percent in weight and color. We continued until Pain was only half a pound and white. He could live with that.

Courage to Speak Calmly: Brody's physical pain finally awakened him to the fact that aggression has real consequences and that his lack of control was creating a vicious cycle. Frustration and embarrassment made him feel stupid and angry. But acting-out made him feel even stupider. His explosions were his poor way of handling stress, but they weren't working. Once he understood this, he was eager to cooperate and keep peace in the family.

Symptoms Persist—But Not for Long: Of course, learning is never a straight march forward. As Brody worked with his new behaviors, old ones snuck back, and so did various physical symptoms. One week he came in coughing and barely able to speak. I suggested that he turn inward and ask what the cough was about. *Guilt* was the culprit. His misbehavior was upsetting him, and he needed to forgive himself for getting so mad. He started to breathe orange *Self-Forgiveness* into his Heart and his hands. Then I suggested he gently use "loving hand energy" to send self-forgiveness into his rasping throat. The anger that was stuck there began to loosen and leave. Soon 95 percent of it was gone. His coughing eased and before long stopped entirely.

Everyone Needs (Animal) Friends: To boost Brody's imagination tool kit, we called in some Animal Friends. Three appeared—Gray Elephant, Silver Fish, and Proud Lion. Elephant agreed to remind Brody of what could calm him. Silver Fish offered a red, white, and blue cooling button. "It's a remote to control my feelings," he explained. "I keep it in my pocket, and it never leaves, even when I change my pants." And Lion gave him *Courage* to face his problems. "It's okay when something goes wrong," Lion told him. "It happens to everyone. Try accepting, and things will work out."

EASY HINTS!

How to be calm around family . . .

BRODY'S TIPS

1 Go outside and breathe calmly.
2 Focus on happier thoughts.
3 Think of the rewards I'll get if I stay calm.
4 Be active—shoot hoops to let out the madness.
5 Tell myself, "I can do it."
6 Use my imagination to create a cartoon version of my family (it'll make me laugh instead of getting mad).
7 Think of what I can do better, then switch my behavior around.

Brody continued to practice his imagination exercises and slowly found new and better ways to express and manage his feelings. When his anger did flair up, he was able to release it through his breath and other Tools. As he put it, "Just by thinking things over and imagining how they could be, I have the ability to not be mad." Brody wanted to include some extra tips (on page 216).

HOW-TO FOR YOU

It wasn't too late for Brody to manage his anger. Now is the time for your child.

⁝⁝ Model Self-Control

You have an enormous influence on how your child handles anger. If you stay calm amid chaos, joke about your own anger, and apologize when you do blow up, your child will often follow your lead. The role model effect is powerful. However, it's not foolproof. Even calm parents, like Brody's, can find themselves face to face with young fury. That's when investigation and imagery are called for.

⁝⁝ Pay Attention to Where Anger Lurks

Anger and its companions—hurt, disappointment, frustration, and betrayal—can hide anywhere in a child's body. Unexpressed, they are emotionally draining, disruptive, and can cause physical pain. Have your child use her imagination to discover where these beastie feelings are stalking. She can then use color or conversation to uncover what would lessen them or hasten their departure.

⁝⁝ Let Body Parts Speak Up

Remind her to connect with the wisdom of her Heart and Belly and any other body part that offers big feelings or wisdom. Anger solutions can come from the most unusual places.

⚉ Wash Away Pain

If stress is causing physical discomfort, employ the Three-Question Exercise (page 117) to help her describe and dissolve her pain. Or suggest a visit to her inner Healing Pond (page 127–128). Soaking in its magical waters can soothe an angry, hurting body.

⚉ Run It Off

Anger generates a lot of energy that physical activity can release. Encourage your child to imagine if she'd prefer to run, swim, jump rope, or dance when she's angry. It will, literally, let off steam. And after she pictures these activities, motivate her to engage in them!

⚉ Invite Guides to Chime In

Remember that Animal Friends, Wizards, and other loving beings are always available to offer counsel and Gifts to cool a hot head. They are tireless, so call on them often.

⚉ Prepare for the Future

Introduce and practice the Tools during times of good behavior, so she'll have an arsenal of positive choices during future upsets. Set up a plan to use simple signals to cue her when stress is high, like making a "b" to remind her to do the Balloon Breath. (Use your right hand, create a circle with your thumb and index finger and hold your middle to pinky fingers up straight.) Or use a funny code word to help her recall how she feels in her Special Place. As she practices, this short-hand system can calm her faster.

⚉ Short-Circuit Anger with Positive Feelings

It's hard to stay mad when you're reliving a joyful moment. When an anger avalanche hits, have her take a cooling time-out, then shift attention to happier images. Point to the Special Place drawing in her room or keep a few photos on hand to evoke a peaceful vacation spot. Even if they only work sometimes, these visual reminders may give her a brief relief from turbulent feelings and increase the likelihood of her calming down.

The Meadow of Peace and Gentleness
An Imagery for Inner Peace

If your child has an issue with anger, or if you'd like her to develop more tranquility, this imagery is a good start. Repeating it daily, for twenty-one to thirty days, will help ensure that she makes it her own. As with other guided journeys, choose whether you'd like to speak the words yourself or use a recording.

Close your eyes and remember your Special Place and how very good you feel there. The memory helps calm you. Now imagine walking on a path made entirely of light . . . it twinkles softly in your favorite color. Notice it under your feet and all around you. The path leads you to a beautiful meadow filled with fragrant flowers and ripe fruit trees. Perhaps there are birds singing in the background or the sound of a fresh running stream nearby . . . you decide, then listen closely. All around you are gently rolling hills in lush shades of green and yellow, purple and pink. The air is a perfect temperature; the sunlight warm. Here you can let go of any hurt, disappointment, frustration, or anger—let go of all your troubles—and be at peace.

Find a comfortable place under a big shade tree. Perhaps there is a chair or blanket waiting for you, or maybe just sit on the soft mossy grass. Relax. You are in The Meadow of Peace and Gentleness. Anything you need to nurture yourself is provided here.

A special box has been waiting for you here for a very long time, hidden underground. It holds the power of peace. Inner peace. Some of your Guides show up to help you unearth it. They may be your Wizard, Animal Friends, or loved ones. Nearby are the shovels and tools you need for uncovering your peace box. You slowly remember that long ago, possibly in your dreams, you planted a seed of peace, which has grown much bigger over time. Allow yourself to dig up the box. You might be surprised at how easily you can bring more peace into your life.

Now open the box. Whatever you planted so long ago is now a Gift to remind you that inner peace is inside you. If you are not sure what it is, or if you don't quite understand it, one of your wise Guides is there to explain. Ask him any questions you have about what you found in the box or how you will use it in your life. Allow yourself to be quiet and listen for anything else your Wizard or Animal Friends want to tell you or that you want to say.

Give yourself a few moments to explore your meadow and to enjoy this very peaceful place inside. Allow any nonpeaceful thoughts or pictures to float away, or release them any way you wish. As you return to your breathing, you return to peace. You deserve each moment to be peaceful and loving. As you breathe, you breathe in peace . . . and love . . . and you let go of any feelings or thoughts you no longer need. You can do this anytime you want.

When you are ready, find yourself once again, walking on your bright path to the center of your Heart. Become aware of your body, your breathing, and where you are. Bring yourself back here, staying very calm, knowing that you will return to this peaceful meadow many times.

CHAPTER 11

Go For the Gold—
Celebrate the Bronze

Achieving Success at School
and in Sports

> I can wash out my rotting
> brain with white foam. After
> I tidy it, my brain feels good
> and I can work better. My
> clean brain is like a flower.
>
> —*Kimberly, age eight*

★ Has your child ever come to you tear-stained and
defeated because she failed a test? Or barricaded
himself in his room because he didn't make the team? Maybe she's
reluctant to return to science class because of a "messed up" project,
or he's afraid to perform in a recital. Academia and sports create such
pressures to win that kids can lose the simple joy of learning and
playing. This seems to start earlier and earlier. Children used to learn
to read in the first grade; now phonics are taught in preschool. Tutoring is on the rise—for smart kids. I see bright six-year-olds stuck in
after-school programs designed to give them "an edge." One nursery
director referred a child to me because he couldn't write his letters . . .
at four! She worried about how he would fare in kindergarten. All I
could think was, "What happened to climbing the jungle gym and
riding a trike?" Children need to develop big muscle skills before the
small ones—those used for drawing and writing—can be trained.

Kids of all ages complain to me about grades. They compare

themselves to their peers and come up lacking; Bs and Cs are rarely acceptable. Even when parents say, "Just do your best," it can be confusing. Children do so much these days—school, sports, music, art, dance, and more—that it's impossible to do their best in everything. Something has to give.

It's the same in sports. While team sports teach many positive qualities—getting along with others, patience, and healthy competition—too much rivalry, especially at a young age, can leach the fun out of any activity. In fact, beloved games can become a source of pain, not play. Six-year-old Jade was crushed because she didn't get a trophy from her T-ball team. The prizes went only to first through fifth place, which left out Jade and three other girls. Palmer, nine, spent most of his time at Little League warming the bench; he couldn't compete with kids who'd played since first grade. Meanwhile, star players on TV make it look so effortless that it's easy for kids (and grown-ups) to forget everyone has to practice and fail in order to play well. Even baseball legend Babe Ruth struck out 1,330 times, and he was already a professional.

Success is wonderful, but winning isn't everything. While physical fitness is critical to healthy growth, teamwork and losing graciously may be as valuable as a trophy. Similarly, reading is only one aspect of a child's early education. From five to seven years old, social and emotional development is every bit as important as the three R's of Reading, wRiting, and aRithmetic.[1] We want to turn naturally curious kids into lifelong learners. Not every child will be a genius or super-athlete, but each can aspire to reach his potential. We might want children to go for the gold—in all their endeavors—but they also need to celebrate the bronze, since life brings an abundance of both. Moreover, we want them to preserve their natural love for "the game," whatever it may be.

Imagery can enrich every performance situation. It helps your child enhance success, accept disappointment, boost confidence, reduce anxiety, and improve motivation.[2] In fact, Olympic athletes and college coaches have been tapping the power of visualization to win games for decades.[3] Competitors mentally rehearse their skills using their senses—imagining what they see, how their bodies feel, what their muscles do, and hearing the cheering crowd. The brain interprets these vivid images as a true physical experience because a visualized practice or performance can engage muscles almost as much as the real thing.[4] One mom I worked with taught her son's entire softball team to improve their game with imagery; not surprisingly they had a winning season.

Imagination is just as effective with schoolwork and creative pursuits. Ten-year-old Reece had difficulty preparing for tests until he visualized a private study hall with a silver desk. As he read his textbooks, the information floated directly from his book into his brain. Eleven-year-old Faith was so scared of failing she was too paralyzed to study, until she envisioned a colorful magic cloud bringing "relaxation and happiness." That helped her go from her bed to her desk, where she started to work. And eight-year-old Stacey managed to turn her fear of choir performances into a source of power. She took the butterflies in her tummy and made them her picture of transformation. A wise Nightingale gifted her with a magical Butterfly Necklace, to remind this budding singer how beautiful and talented she was.

In this chapter, we'll see how imagination can solve performance problems. You'll learn not only how to help your child do his best in school, sports, and other areas, but how to address the natural setbacks and disappointments that come with risk taking. Whatever your child's strengths and weaknesses, the Nine Tools will help him fulfill his potential and brave new challenges as he shoots for his dreams.

If I'm So Smart, Why Is Learning So Hard?

Making the Best of What You Have

Kimberly was a brilliant eight-year-old with learning issues. She was smarter than 98 percent of her peers, yet she had difficulty reading and writing. She became extremely self-critical and thought herself "stupid." Her kindergarten teacher had noticed Kimberly had trouble with directions and needed tasks broken down step by step. He recommended tutoring, but the idea of a five-year-old needing a tutor so shocked her parents, they let it go. However, they sought help when Kimberly continued writing letters and words backward in third grade. In addition to tutoring and special school services, Kimberly's parents felt her artistic nature would benefit from art therapy and imagery support. They made a good decision.

All children learn differently. And while we want them to enjoy learning as they earn good grades, few schools accommodate the full range of educational styles. Traditional schoolrooms emphasize an auditory approach: the teacher talks; the kids listen. This effectively leaves out visual kids who need to "see" the material, tactile ones who discover by touch, and kinesthetic children who move while learning something new. This is not about preference; their brains actually work differently.

One simple explanation uses the popular "left brain/right brain" model: Kids with a dominant "left" brain do well with verbal/auditory instruction. They learn to read by sounding out words and tend to be logical, linear thinkers. Children with a more developed "right" brain are comfortable with visual and intuitive information. Sounding out words can be challenging, and they often read more easily with a whole word approach. Some kids seem to live in their bodies more than their brains. They need to move—jump or tap their feet or fingers—in order to concentrate and remember. Others need extra stimulation.

They study well with music or television on in the background but lose focus in a "quiet, boring" classroom. These kids are as motivated to learn as their auditory classmates, yet schools often label them slow, lazy, and, in the case of kinesthetic kids, disruptive. Without understanding and support, their work and self-esteem can suffer.

Imagery creates a safe place to honor and harness a child's learning style. By engaging the imagination and emotions, the Nine Tools can reduce stress, remove obstacles, and improve concentration and retention. That's what I was counting on with Kimberly.

Kimberly came in frustrated. She had once enjoyed school, but as each grade became more demanding, she felt she was back-pedaling and had forgotten what she'd already learned. She lacked confidence and was uncomfortable raising her hand to ask questions or answer them. It took her more than four hours to complete an hour's worth of homework. And she felt her parents expected too much of her. Sometimes she'd fake illness to skip class.

Parental Support Is Not Always Enough: Kimberly's parents did what they could. Her mom helped with homework and, when that failed, found an excellent tutor. The school resource specialist also consulted with Kimberly's teachers and provided extra, small group support. But all this special help backfired. Kimberly was stressed by the time commitments, additional work, and what seemed like an even greater pressure to succeed. She told me she still felt stupid and wondered if her brain had simply rotted.

Worry Warps the Brain: After a few Balloon Breaths, Kimberly closed her eyes, turned inward, and took a look at her brain. It was filled with compartments: a blue area for homework, a sad gray part, a bright yellow dancing stage, and a happy red section because a holiday was approaching. We focused on clearing out all the gloomy bits in her brain and scrubbing away negative thoughts about learning and homework. Kimberly also spiffed up the alert and focused places so she could remember what she learned. "I can wash out my rotting brain with white foam," she realized. "After I tidy it, my brain feels good and I can work better. My clean brain is like a flower." Kimberly wound up with an "awesome happy brain" that helped her complete her homework more easily and accurately.

But Kimberly still had another complaint. Pressure about success affected her sleep.

Face Monster Pressure: Every night, as Kimberly closed her eyes, a space alien interrupted her sleepy-time thoughts. "He comes into my room from the corner," she explained, "so I don't want to close my eyes. He's green and looks slimy with lumps and bumps." I asked if she knew who this creepy guy was: "What part of you does he represent?" Without hesitation, Kimberly replied, "My anger and sadness."

Let Your Feelings Speak: In her desire to be good girl, good student, and good daughter, Kimberly had kept her anger and sadness bottled up. They now spilled out as a monster that wrecked her restful nights. "Why?" I asked, and Kimberly exploded. "'Cause his life is too hard! After school he has hard homework. He never gets to relax. He always wakes up early for tutoring, and he misses the easy stuff at school. He wants to play with his friends. He never does anything fun. He wants two hours of free time every day."

....

Backtrack Alert
....

Kimberly had made progress when she connected the alien to her anger and sadness. But instead of continuing with her own feelings, she went back to the monster. Had she lost ground? Absolutely not! Of course, "he" is Kimberly. It's often less threatening for children to separate

themselves from big feelings. It doesn't stop the process. Not only is it okay to work in symbols and metaphors, it can actually be useful.
....

Negotiate with the Enemy: Two hours of free time each day seemed impossible; there was too much for Kimberly to do. I asked if the alien was willing to compromise. He was, and agreed to sixty minutes, but Kimberly didn't know if she could find even this hour. She needed assistance.

Time-Management Wizard Arrives: I suggested Kimberly consider Wizard Wisdom, and a Time-Management Wizard showed up. He wore robes covered with orange suns and yellow moons, had a long beard, lots of wrinkles, and long bony fingers that held a golden staff. His Gift for Kimberly was a special CD, *The Magic of Time.* It had tracks like "Setting up priorities," "How to get things done," and "What to do with spare time." Whenever a new problem arose, a new solution appeared on the CD. With this input, Kimberly was able to find one free hour a day. In fact, by counting drive time with her mom, she almost reached that two-hour mark. She also resolved to speak up and see how Mom could help lighten her load.

Spelling Wizard from Planet X: Kimberly was so enthralled with her Time Wizard, she requested additional guides. Spelling was a huge stumbling block. Kimberly had been misspelling twenty-five words on paragraph dictations and felt discouraged. Enter the Spelling Wizard. He had a big head—"cause he's so smart"—and promised to help her remember the words she studied. His message: "Have fun with your spelling. Turn it into a game." With Spelling Wizard at her side, coaching her for each week's quiz, the task felt more like fun than a chore. Her scores began to improve a little each week; soon, she was down to just three or four errors.

Let Albert Einstein Be Your Guide: Kimberly then asked for a Math Wizard. Albert Einstein showed up, wearing addition, subtraction, and multiplication tables on his clothes. Kimberly resonated with Einstein's early life. Her dad told her that he had been considered dumb as a boy but, of course, turned out to be a genius. That cheered her considerably. Wizard Albert told her: "Just take your time; it's not a contest. Do belly breathing. It'll help you stay calm enough to remember what you know. You can do this."

QUICK TIP!   Wizards Are Perfect Tutors

When learning is challenging, Wizard Wisdom is the best guide. Animal Friends offer protection, insight, and gifts, but Wizards are magical teachers whose powers can transform brains. At least in your child's imagination.

Kimberly took advantage of a variety of Wizards to help her with schoolwork, and added Report and Reading Wizards. She became more open to resources her parents and school made available and was able to accommodate her learning style in a regular class. And she found time to enjoy her many creative talents—dance, painting, sculpting, and ceramics.

HOW-TO FOR YOU

Kimberly maximized her brainpower with her imagination skills. Your child can do the same.

❚❚ Pay Attention to School Worries

Listen to your child's thoughts and concerns about school. Ask him about his favorite subjects—What are the easiest?

The hardest? Are the more challenging subjects the ones he likes least? How would he like school to be? Have him visualize what he desires. Don't let homework overshadow emotions. Sharing his dreams and feelings will bring you closer.

❖ Hunt Down Resources

Ask what resources your school offers children with different learning styles. If your child doesn't qualify for "special services," there may be reading clinics, homework labs, or teachers who stay late. Keep searching for what you need. If private tutoring isn't an option, consider college kids who need teaching experience.

❖ Refresh the Brain

Encourage your child to take time before homework to center himself and clear his fuzzy brain of negative thoughts about his abilities or the subject at hand. Have him start Balloon Breathing, then imagine cleaning his brain with foam, light, or any other substance that pops up. He can picture his brain primed to learn, or increase his brainpower with a *Super Smart Solution*. Finish by having him imagine how satisfied he'll feel when he successfully completes his homework.

❖ Give Tests a Positive Spin

Have your child imagine the grade he hopes for at the top of a returned test. Suggest he picture the smile on his teacher's face when she hands it to him. This is not hocus-pocus. Visualizing a good grade will reinforce his goal and encourage him to work hard to achieve it. The rewards for clear goals and hard work are practical magic.

❖ Celebrate Improvement

Not every arrow hits the mark. Help your child acknowledge small successes and recognize subtle victories along the way to an improved score—it's a critical part of maturation. It's great to get the gold, but every outcome offers opportunities and lessons. Each improvement is a small victory.

Get Set for Next Time

You can use disappointments to prepare and motivate your child for future success. Listen to how he feels about his achievement. Let him know you understand by repeating back what he's told you—using his words or your own. Your empathy will go a long way. Ask what he liked about how he prepared—for example, how he studied for the test—and how he'd like it to be next time. Brainstorm and fine-tune what he needs to do better. Together, set a goal, write it down, and ask what help he needs from you to achieve it.

Reduce Pressure

Preparation relieves worry. Get a poster-sized calendar, break down assignments into smaller bits, and develop a plan. A book report due next month can be divided like this: Read ten pages a day (for a 150-page book), use five days to take notes, five to write the draft, then five more to polish. Have your child visualize finishing with days to spare. Color code by subject (Science—green; English—yellow) or type of assignment (tests—red; homework—blue).

Reduce Pressure Some More

Figure out together how to reduce his work and social load. Maybe this isn't the time to study piano, with all the practice it requires, or perhaps two sports teams are too much. By preserving the activities he loves, and letting go of extra commitments, you free up his time and energy for calmer study and better performance all around.

⁑ Use Wizards for All Subjects

Your child may have an all-purpose Wizard, but he might also succeed with specific Wizards. Call in a Spelling, Math, or Science Wizard. Ask for help, and follow his wisdom.

Public Panic

Overcoming Performance Jitters

Six-year-old Leo was a funny and friendly guy. He had loads of buddies and was always cracking them up with his crazy impressions. His parents were in creative fields—Mom was a costume designer, Dad a writer—and though they never pushed their son, he loved to dress up and entertain the family. Their home was often filled with roaring laughter at the impromptu plays Leo and his siblings put on. So when the holiday school pageant came around, Leo's teacher asked him to introduce the show, and everyone thought he would shine.

So did Leo . . . at first. But once rehearsals started on stage, he froze. He suddenly realized that the auditorium would be filled with strangers. And while it was obvious to all that Leo was a born showman, he couldn't handle the internal pressure. He lost all his confidence, started to cry, and ran to the bathroom, embarrassed. His anxiety turned into horrible stomach pains. They started to attack when he read aloud in class. His wise pediatrician realized that the best course of treatment wasn't medication, but meditation. So he sent Leo to me.

Sometimes kids are so afraid of speaking in front of a group that they don't even try. Public speaking is the number one fear among people of all ages;[5] it even tops fear of dying. A child who seems shy, stubborn, rebellious, or indifferent may actually suffer from a deep fear of failure or a belief that she's not good enough. Leo is a perfect example of how worry inhibits functioning, and how imagination can release that pressure, freeing a child to face all kinds of "performance" situations.

Start Slow: When I met Leo, his dread of speaking in public sent him into near panic. These overwhelming feelings prevented him from thinking or acting rationally, so we started slowly with gentle breathing. To shift the attention from his worry cycle, I suggested he concentrate on his Heart. When he could refocus to a calmer place, I knew he'd be able to find his own answers—and believe in them.

QUICK TIP!

Use a Variation of the Balloon Breath

"Heart-Centered" Script

"Breathe very slowly. That's right. Breath in and out . . . in and out . . . sending your breath two to three inches below your navel. Focus on your Heart Center, the area in the middle of your chest. Place your hand over your Heart Center, allowing yourself to be comforted. As you breathe, put your awareness there."

This is a great way to shift your child's attention from her worried head-brain into her calmer heart-brain. The physical touch can also bring great comfort.

Create a "Problem" Picture: Leo described his upsetting stomach pain as black and gray, "a little squiggle that's like a monster that scares me. There's lightning inside that spreads out and makes me more nervous."

Ask for Help Right Away: Leo's distress required immediate relief. I suggested he ask his "monster pain" what color would be calming to breathe in. He chose orange, and to his surprise, it helped. By slowly breathing in the color orange, Leo soothed his belly.

Find a Safe Place: Once we soothed the acute pain, we focused on Leo's performance worries by having him imagine a Special Place. He created an imaginary garden playground with a stage built for two. His best friend was with him, laughing and swaying on nearby swings. The stage, decorated with a winter holiday backdrop, awaited them with everything needed for rehearsing: costumes, makeup, and the script. Here, in his sunny mental sanctuary, Leo worked through his concerns by practicing with his friend, gaining the confidence he needed to get up in front of a large group in the real world and speak the words he had memorized.

Hang Your Worries Out to Dry: Leo was making much progress, yet some residual worry remained. I asked him what picture came to help and, when nothing arose, suggested that he hang his thoughts and worries in a colorful sack outside his Special Place. He could pick them up later if he wanted them back. Doing so allowed him a respite from his mind worries, reducing their fearful noise so that he could actually hear his intuition.

Backtrack Alert

Sometimes kids just don't "see" an image. That's fine. We all get information differently. Sometimes we think it, or feel it, or hear it. And sometimes nothing comes. If that happens, simply ask a few questions, like does he *sense* the *Courage* to speak in his body somewhere, or can he imagine *telling* himself that he can do this? If he still draws a blank, just stop for now and try again another day. Some imaginations take time to warm up.

Meet Your Wizard: Leo's personal Wizard also came through to offer wise counsel. He had glasses, a long beard, and wore typical

Wizard garb: royal blue gown and tall hat covered with stars. He reminded Leo to "breathe and stay calm," while cheering him on that he "could do it."

Leo and I worked together until he was completely confident of his Imagination Wisdom. Although he opted out of the winter play, by the end of the school year he was back on stage, front and center. Here is his self-instruction for "not losing it" when speaking in public. His simple, yet clear, grasp of the imagery Tools may help your child.

> **EASY HINTS!**
>
> How to stay calm and not freak out at the school play . . .
>
> **LEO'S LIST**
> 1 Do my Balloon Breath.
> 2 Remember how I feel in my Special Place.
> 3 Talk to my (inner) helpers.
> 4 Notice Gifts from my Wizard that help me.
> 5 Talk to my Heart and "gut."
> 6 Remember to tell myself, "I can do it. I am calm."
> 7 Draw my scared feelings so I don't keep them inside.
> 8 Practice, practice, practice.

HOW-TO FOR YOU

The Tools that helped Leo can relieve your child's performance worries.

❊ Focus on the Heart

Ease your child through her anxiety with short simple questions. Start by focusing on her Heart and ask:

- What would soothe your Heart?
- What is it really worried about?
- What does it tell you is best for you?
- How does it tell you to help yourself?

❖ Go to a Safe Special Place

Engage your child in creating an imaginary sanctuary where she can escape the pressure to excel, practice, and build the courage to speak in front of the class, face that recital, or perform in a play.

❖ Provide Relief from Worries

Have her request inner guidance for immediate performance relief. If nothing comes—perhaps from anxiety about the process itself—it's okay to give her a gentle start. Suggest hanging her worries outside or imagining her fears floating away in balloons. Your assistance may inspire her and set her back on track to wisdom within.

❖ Look for Wizard Insight

When stage fright becomes powerful, suggest she summon her inner Wizard—either an all-purpose one or a specialist. She can request magic or notice what Gifts are offered to help worries disappear.

❖ Make a Chart

Advise her to write down which Tools work. Try an erasable white board for easy updates. Review the chart to gently remind her of what she really knows inside whenever she feels overwhelmed or forgets her strengths.

Sports Success

How to Handle Pressure and Still Have Fun

Sassy and sensitive Owen, nine, loved to play soccer more than anything in the world. He had been kicking a ball since he was three and practiced with his dad almost every weekend. But when it came to trying out for the soccer team, he couldn't do it. His lack of confidence prevented him from stepping on the field. He had missed the initial tryouts, and there were only a few more makeup sessions to go. He needed a quick fix—and soon!

Sometimes anxiety can stop kids from engaging in activities they absolutely adore. Love—of a sport, a subject, or an art form—can create unrealistic expectations, an irrational sense of "be good or give up." Parents are often dumbfounded. What happened to the happy child who loved to swim, dance, or play the piano? Who couldn't wait to show off some new trick or lesson? She's still there, but she's lost in a battle between passion and perfection, locked in a struggle that is anything but fun.

Fortunately, Imagination Tools are the perfect way to relieve pressure and restore a sense of play and accomplishment. Owen's mind got him into this state; his imagination could get him out.

Deep Breathing Always Helps: I asked Owen to start his Balloon Breath and focus inward. We concentrated on the fear that kept him from moving forward and the feeling that could help him the most— *Confidence.* It turned out that both were inside his Heart. *Fear* was a saturated black blob—a 7 on the 0 to 10 Scale, and Confidence, a much smaller, green circle, was down to 3.

Fear Aids Confidence with a Chat: A quick conversation seemed to shift the scene. Fear spoke to Confidence. "I know I should go, but I'm scared," it confessed. "But if I don't try, I really won't be able to get on the soccer team." Confidence replied: "I know you want to go. Take me along, I'll help." After a pause, Fear told Confidence, "I'm glad I told you how I felt." Just sharing made a difference.

Fear Versus Confidence—Round Two: I asked Owen to focus on the confidence in his Heart and see how large he could make it with his intention and his breath. Confidence grew into a bright green ball—a 10—way bigger than Fear, which had shrunk to a mere 1 or 1½. Once Owen mastered this crisis in faith, he tried out and made the team.

It's Not Over Yet: I thought we were done, but six months later, Owen returned. He was having trouble with his coach, who screamed and intimidated rather than give positive encouragement. He had seen Coach use a laser stare and sharp tongue to pulverize a number of his teammates. Owen had a strong sense of fairness and had always cooperated with his instructors. Coach's behavior seemed extremely unfair. And his constant yelling scared the wits out of him. After a tough day at practice, Owen would come home crying. At least once a week, the left side of his head would pound as if a ball were hitting it for hours.

Don't Quit What You Love: Coach's behavior disturbed Owen so much that he stopped trying on the field, and his game suffered. In fact, when his parents brought him back to me, Owen was ready to quit the sport he loved and the team he had worked so hard to join. "I give it my all, and he still yells at me," he lamented. His mom suggested that he tell Coach he was doing his best and ask him not to yell, but he couldn't do that—at least not yet.

Fear in the Heart, Anger in the Knees: Owen knew he was scared of facing Coach. Black Fear returned—this time in his Heart, where love would normally be. I had him check inside his body for what else was lurking. Red *Anger* was hiding in his legs—the very legs he used to run across the soccer field.

Use Three Positives to Overcome Two Negatives: What could help Owen overcome his anxiety and develop the confidence he needed to speak up? We called on *Calm*, *Brave*, and *Loving* feelings. Calm because he needed to be centered to think straight. Brave because he needed the courage to face Coach. And Love to help open his Heart to Coach's point of view and soften the way Owen approached him.

Following a now-familiar routine, we looked for these "good guy" feelings inside. This time, Owen's Calm feelings were a placid sea blue—and mostly in his head with some bits in his arms. His Brave feelings were strong and brown in his feet, especially the left foot, which, coincidentally, led his steps onto the field. Love was down in his Belly (because Fear had taken over his Heart); it was silver, like a medal he treasured.

Talk to Your Feelings: Each feeling held important information about approaching Coach. Fear didn't want to get hurt. Calm reminded Owen that Coach was pretty nice off the soccer field; he might consider speaking to him away from practice. Brave let Owen know there was nothing to worry about since Coach wouldn't actually hurt him. Brave also gave Owen a Gift: a water bottle filled with special liquid he could drink to increase his courage. And Love made everything seem lighter and smaller.

With all this feeling advice, Owen practiced what he wanted to say and imagined a positive outcome. It paid off. He spoke up from a centered place and clearly told Coach

---

EASY HINTS!

How to face a "crazed" coach . . .

OWEN'S OPUS

1 Take five to ten deep breaths, four times a day.
2 Use color to adjust my feelings.
3 Imagine myself doing well and Coach complimenting me (once a day for two minutes).
4 Imagine talking to Coach and telling him how I feel, and Coach changing his behavior (one to two times a day).
5 Listen to my relaxation CD (every night for a month).

how it upset him when he yelled. So much so that he wanted to quit. He didn't understand why Coach couldn't just talk in a regular tone. Much to Owen's astonishment, Coach was grateful that he had come to him. He had wondered why Owen had been retreating. Now they could focus on—and enjoy—their mutual love of soccer.

Owen was thrilled with the outcome. His notes on what else worked for him appear on page 238.

HOW-TO FOR YOU

If Owen could find the courage to try out for his favorite team sport, play his heart out, get shot down, confront his coach, and continue to play like a champ, surely your child can.

✂ Face Feelings

Help your child get in touch with whatever feelings are holding her back from participating in the activities she used to love. Have her close her eyes and look inside, scanning from the top of her head to the tips of her toes. As she thinks about the task at hand, what feelings seem to "light up?" *Fear? Worry? Anxiety? Failure?* What colors are they? What shapes or images do they suggest? Just naming stuck emotions can bring enormous relief.

✂ Have a Heart to Heart

Once she identifies feelings that help or hinder her performance, suggest a Heart to Heart conversation with them. She can ask them what they want to tell her, what might calm them down, or what she needs to understand in order to feel better and perform with ease. With honesty and respect, she and her emotional obstacles can work out a resolution to any conflict.

⠏ Use Intention to Turn the Tide

Let your child's positive intention of enjoying or excelling in her sport or art form turn around the situation. Suggest she think about being confident—or any other quality that is important to her—and breathe that color into negative feelings. See if she can fill her entire body with the good feelings. If she can, worry will often step aside.

⠏ Boost Confidence with Imagery Practice

Ask your child how she visualizes her accomplishment. Is she skating figure eights? Hitting a home run? Dancing a solo? Playing a concerto? Whether she tends to see, hear, or feel images, help her develop vivid imagination pictures that include as many senses as possible, and in real time. Practicing for five minutes, two to three times a day, in advance and right before the event, will increase her confidence and her performance.

⠏ Engage Positive Language

In visualization, perspective doesn't matter—she can feel herself inside the experience or watch it like a movie. But language does. Help her use affirmations in her performance images. The creative brain can't register negative instructions. "Don't miss that note!" can be interpreted as "Miss that note!" "I can hit that note!" works much better.

⠏ Put Your Knowledge into Practice

Help your child identify priorities. Does she want to go for the gold, silver, or bronze? Does she want to play competitively or for recreation? She may not want to be the best, or even *her* best. Maybe she's just looking for fun, without competition. Any answer is right because it's hers. What matters most is that she does what she loves.

Climbing a Mountain of Success
Imagery for Accomplishment

As you focus on your breathing, imagine yourself walking on a path in a beautiful meadow. There's a forest to your right, open space to your left, and a tall mountain ahead in the distance. Out of the forest comes a wise and loving Animal Friend. Notice what kind of animal it is—what it looks and smells like. Together, you will climb the mountain. It looks huge, but you have a feeling you'll be successful. Your Animal Friend tells you not to worry, and you don't.

When you reach the base of the mountain, there are many roads up ahead. Find the path that's right for you. Tools and supplies are waiting—a hiking stick, shovel, food, water, anything you need. Your Animal Friend carries them all.

As you find your way up the mountain, your path begins to curve and feel a little more difficult. Perhaps it gets steep or looks rocky. Maybe the sun is setting, and you feel cold. A soft light streams down from the mountain to warm you and help you find your way.

You ask your Animal Friend for advice. He suggests you stop at a nearby cave. A gold star floats out of the cave and, before your eyes, turns into a Wizard. Your Personal Wizard. What does he or she look like? How is he or she dressed? Ask your Wizard any question about your journey. And listen patiently for the answer. Whatever your mountain may be—doing well in school, being the best athlete you can be, singing in front of an audience—your Wizard can offer advice on how to reach your goal. And Gifts! Watch as your Wizard pulls out a Gift to inspire you and help you to reach the top. You might be surprised by what it is. Keep the Gift with you for the rest of your trip up the mountain.

Take a little time to rest. When you're ready, continue your journey. Pay attention to what's around you. As you near the top, notice how the paths all come together. See the clearing at the very, very top. Step into it. You did it! Feel how proud and thrilled you are to have climbed this massive mountain. How successful. Maybe you thought you couldn't do it, but now you know you can. You can do whatever you set out to do. Look around. There are many other mountains to climb someday. All will be part of your continuing success. And you always have help. Your Wizard, your Animal Friends, and many others will be there for you.

Now notice the shape of a figure in the distance. As you get closer, realize this person is kind, loving, and generous—an incredible, wise wonderful being. You can feel the love. The figure starts to come into clear view and you realize that person is really . . . the best parts of you. Come closer—with your arms outstretched. And hug each other, taking in the best of You.

When you are ready, come back down the mountain any way you like. Come down, down to the very bottom, down to the meadow. Remember, each time you climb this and other mountains, you will learn something new. Say good-bye to your Wizard and Animal Friend for now. Take time to walk through the meadow on your own, remembering who you are and what you can achieve. Take all the time you need. Then return to your path and bring yourself back here.

CHAPTER 12

Can't We All Just Get Along?

Be kind to other people, and they will treat you like you want.

—Andy, age six

Living Peacefully with Siblings, Friends, and Parents

★ All eight-year-old Lara wanted from her big brother was peace. She hated arguing over TV and was hurt and angry at his constant teasing. Seven-year-old Miriam cried herself to sleep every night. Last year's friends wound up in another class, and she felt isolated. Eleven-year-old Dalton kept landing in parental hot water. He thought he was a big kid now and resisted their strict rules.

Kids want positive interactions with friends and family, but buttons get pushed, defenses go up, and friction abounds. Or they withdraw into loneliness and isolation. Either way, it's problematic. The single best predictor for a child's success is not IQ, grades, or classroom behavior, but relationships. Those who can't sustain close friendships are at risk for low self-esteem, poor emotional health, and academic difficulties.[1] In fact, a Stanford study found a connection between good social skills and good reading scores in early grades.[2] It's not surprising. Kids who work poorly with classmates and teachers feel left out and sour on school, so learning suffers. Children who enjoy gratifying relationships flourish.

Not that your child must be a social butterfly. Some kids are shy, and others are content with one or two good friends. It's the quality of the friendships, not the quantity, that matters. Not what kind of friends she has, but the kind of friend she is.[3]

You play a crucial role. Cooperation, empathy, kindness, fair play, and self-control don't always come naturally to children; they are skills, taught through practice, just like making a bed and riding a bike. One of the best ways to help your child learn them is to model them. Kids are great imitators. If you want to encourage kindness and generosity, let them see yours. To foster self-control, watch how you respond to frustration and anger. Empathy—the ability to imagine what others are feeling—can be challenging. But if you share your feelings, let your kids express theirs, and encourage them to consider others, most will learn it.

Play is another important way children learn to relate to others. The games and squabbles they get into with siblings, neighbors, and classmates are boot camp for social skills. The backyard and the schoolyard create constant learning opportunities for following directions, listening, creative problem solving, standing up for themselves, and fairness.

But some children need more instruction. Perhaps they're only children without siblings to practice on, maybe a baby brother has thrown old ways into question, or a new school has sparked inappropriate behavior. Possibly it's just the next stage in development; every year presents children with change, new challenges, and new social demands. Each conflict is a learning opportunity. And your child's imagination is a great study partner. It gives a clear picture of her struggle and a safe place to practice better responses.

Whatever kids visualize and mentally rehearse, they are more likely to actualize in life. Six-year-old Alec was so shy he couldn't ask anyone in the schoolyard to play with him until he breathed in royal blue *Confidence*, and black *Doubt* disintegrated. Ten-year-old Melody couldn't stand up to her big sister, who always took advantage of her good nature, until a Wizard coached her to say "No" in a strong, clear voice. And nine-year-old Jenna had so many issues with her family, they felt like "aliens" to her. She went to outer space for answers. The "little people" she met on an imagined planet gave her a gold locket with a picture of her parents hugging her—a reminder they really did love her.

This chapter explores how imagination can teach children to cooperate with others. By starting inside the family, your child can develop emotional intelligence that organically extends to friends and peers.

The Slimy Green Eyes of Jealousy

Help for Sibling Rivalry

Nine-year-old Taylor's jealousy of her four-year-old brother caused angry tears at home. Although she had longed for a sibling, it was different once Riley arrived. Taylor flip-flopped between loving hugs and dangerous squeezing, between helping change the baby and ignoring him. While her parents had expected ambivalence at first, they were stunned to be dealing with it three years later. When Taylor accidentally dunked the little boy in the neighbor's pool, and he cried whenever she approached, they decided intervention was needed.

Nearly every only child I see dreams of having siblings. And almost all kids who have them wish, at some point, they didn't. After all, getting along with siblings can be tough. Little kids fight over toys. Big ones tease and criticize. All children compete for their parents' attention. And admit it or not, they compare themselves: who does more chores or enjoys more privileges, which one is better at school or sports. No matter what you do to keep peace, your kids are guaranteed to drive each other crazy. Sibling rivalry is an inevitable part of growing up.[4] And paradoxically, that's good news.

Brothers and sisters often provide a child's first opportunity to develop important social skills such as sharing, taking turns, and resolving conflicts. With your guidance, they can also learn honesty, kindness, and tolerance. In fact, kindergarteners who have one or more siblings get along better with classmates than do only children.[5] To sail the stormy seas of rivalry, teach your kids to work together. Imagery and deep listening enable them to express the complex feelings that siblings set off and give them a safe way to explore new behavior. Previewing change in their imagination makes it easier to shift behavior in the world. That's what happened with Taylor.

Taylor States Her Case: Taylor was a tangle of complaints and mixed feelings. She felt replaced by her brother. He got the lion's share of her parents' time, could do no wrong, and was a nuisance in her life. Yet she still wanted to play with him. She couldn't understand why he avoided her. She hadn't meant to hurt him; she loved Riley. But she was also angry and confused. And because she couldn't see the connection between her behavior and his reaction, she just sank into a mad, bad mood.

Picture of Pressure: Taylor also felt pressure from her parents to be the "good big sister," a role she hadn't bargained for. The burden was too great. Wondering what her stress felt like, I asked her to go inside to create a picture. An image came immediately. A huge tree had fallen and landed across her chest. She could barely breathe.

Elephant to the Rescue: I suggested Taylor close her eyes and imagine someone, perhaps an Animal buddy, helping her. She saw an Elephant wrapping its trunk around the tree, lifting it off her and tossing it away. The relief was palpable as Taylor let out a deep sigh.

Ambivalence Has Its Place: I assured Taylor that it was normal to have all kinds of feelings for her brother. We considered positive and negative emotions. She closed her eyes, and I asked her to imagine where inside her body she kept these strong feelings and what they looked like.

Accept the Good and Bad: Taylor easily found "loving feelings" in her Heart, but she had a harder time with negative ones. She believed it was terrible to have bad thoughts about anyone, though clearly, from her behavior, she had them. Given permission to look at her real feelings, Taylor discovered *Hate* hiding in her little fingers, which curled into a fiery ball. She turned these extremes into characters. She drew *Love* as a smiling red heart with arms and legs, while Hate was a miserable, blue fist-shaped being. Now we had something to work with.

Love Hits a Snag: I suggested Taylor use her breath to send red Love for Riley throughout her body to transform her hateful feelings. She was able to send love everywhere except her fingers, where the bad feelings lived. Love couldn't penetrate this closed door and just bounced off. More work was required.

Hate Reveals Its Source: A week later, the bad feelings were still there, but when Taylor tuned in, *Sad* had replaced Hate. She was now in touch with what was really going on. She cried about not being the youngest anymore and how she hardly got any notice. She felt left out.

Call In Mr. Magic: We decided to ask Taylor's fingers what would open the door so Love could soothe her Sad feelings. Again, she found the answer inside: "For me to be nicer to my brother and for him to be nicer to me." Bam! She made the connection between her behavior and Riley's response. But how could she accomplish this?

She needed advice big-time. I wondered if a Wizard might do the trick. Enter Mr. Magic. He gave her an exquisite perfume bottle filled with potent medicine. She was to sprinkle some on herself and her brother every morning. Now she could imagine sending love from her Heart to her Sad little fingers. Nothing would stop those good feelings from spreading.

Find Confidence to Speak Up for What You Want: There was one step left. Taylor had to tell her parents when she needed more attention. She was afraid they would be mad, but she knew if she didn't ask, she'd take out her anger on Riley. Purple tears of *Fear* popped up in her Belly when she thought about asking for what she wanted. Where could she find *Confidence*? It glowed near her Heart, a little to the left. By breathing its golden color into Belly's purple Fear, her nerves shifted and certainty arrived. She was ready to negotiate.

Blue Bird of Advice: Bird Friends gave additional insight into "the brother situation." Taylor imagined a typical argument—how annoying Riley was when he came in her room and "messed with" her things. Her frustration was so flagrant, she plotted revenge. But before she could get a good plan going, I asked if an Animal Friend might offer assistance. Blue Bird flew in with suggestions: instead of punching him or pulling hair, maybe she could punch and pull her pillow. Or if he was bugging her in the car, she might ignore him by singing—but not so loud as to get in trouble.

Plan B: Taylor liked Blue Bird's ideas, but they didn't always work. "I'm trying to stop punching him," she explained one day. "I know I have to. But I can't. And I yell before I hit him." So we switched to Plan B and called back Mr. Magic. This time he offered her the Gift of a *Magic Peach* to control her aggression and help her to listen to her Heart. "When you eat it, you think about other things so you don't focus on your brother bothering you. It'll be like he's not even there."

Red Bird Cleans Up: Taylor realized she felt physically ill after these fights—as if all the bad feelings between them landed right back on her. She took some deep breaths and went inside to see if someone could help out. That's when Red Bird showed up and started pecking the sticky feelings off her back. Red Bird even managed to catch some bits before they clung to her. There were, however, a few bad feelings that even he couldn't get. And some part of Taylor knew why. "He can only get rid of stuff my brother is putting on me," she blurted out. "But stuff I'm putting on myself . . . only I can fix." Quite a responsible insight for nine! She was finally able to imagine sending love to Riley and receiving good feelings back.

Baby Talk Intrudes: Once Taylor got past her anger, one last issue arose. Sometimes she'd come into my office babbling baby talk and wanting to play with preschool toys. When I wondered how old she felt, she said four. "Who else is four?" I asked. She smiled slyly and murmured, "Riley," adding, "At home I get noticed more this way." She clearly needed better self-soothing strategies.

Relearn Self-Love: Taylor was a perfect candidate for the *Loving Yourself from Day One* imagery (Chapter 5). As she closed her eyes and did her Balloon Breath, I asked if she could imagine herself as a baby. She pictured being held, loved, and receiving all the attention she craved, in every way she wanted. A big smile came to her now peaceful face. I brought her slowly through the years to her present age, but we didn't stop there. I suggested she imagine moving forward into the future and

---

EASY HINTS!

To be nicer to my brother . . .

TAYLOR'S TRICKS

1 Check in with my Heart and fingers.
2 Talk to my Wizard, Mr. Magic.
3 Use the medicine and Gifts I receive.
4 Use Balloon Breath as needed.
5 Use different colors to heal bad feelings.
6 Speak up! Say how I feel and ask for what I need.

growing strong, healthy, and happy. She could do that, and vowed to listen regularly to the tape I made her. It felt good to take care of herself this way, and she was soon able to let Riley be the baby and become the real big sister. Taylor shared what worked best for her on page 249.

HOW-TO FOR YOU

Taylor used her imagination to sort out her complex feelings toward her little brother. You can use similar approaches for sibling squabbles in your home.

Don't Underestimate Stress

When pressure is high, patience for sibling shenanigans drops. Teach your child to use the 0 to 10 Scale for stress check-ups, then use Balloon Breathing and other imagery Tools to lower reactivity and raise tolerance.

Find Out What's Under Those Big Bad Feelings

Start by accepting and validating whatever your child is feeling about his sibling. Then gently guide him to the core issue. Listen to whatever image he offers for angry or hateful feelings, then say, "Now close your eyes, and be surprised at what's under . . . [the big bad feeling]." When he faces the emotions under his distress, he will be closer to understanding how to release them and make peace with his sis or bro.

Work Those Animal Guides

Have your child call in animal advice for any sibling disputes. Old Animal Friends might return, or new ones may appear.

Use Wizard Wisdom in a Pinch

Animal Friends may solve only part of the sibling rivalry problem. Don't hesitate to have your child ask for a Wizard or two. They usually provide a plan.

❖ Have Feelings Talk to Each Other

Your child probably has a range of emotions about his siblings, some of which are as distinct as love/hate or happy/mad. Having his feelings "speak" to each other can result in a creative compromise. Once they get the hang of it, kids of similar age can practice this together, as the *Anger* of one negotiates with the *Sadness* of the other. But that comes later, after each has learned tolerance for his own hard feelings.

❖ Unique, Not Equal

It's okay to treat your kids differently. They are different ages and have different personalities and needs. For instance, a ten-year-old may be allowed to stay up later than a five-year-old. Soccer practices might simply be more frequent than dance recitals, although you love attending both. Talk to your children about how and why you make these choices. Listen to any hurt feelings, and let them know what you can change, what you can't, and why. At the same time, try to avoid favoritism and comparisons. Celebrate each child's uniqueness, and encourage cooperation, not competition.

Friendship Frenzy

Getting Along with Peers

Seven-year-old Freddie was a misfit at school. Every day he complained: "It's boring." "The girls are bossy." "The boys pick on me." All true. But underneath it all, Freddie wanted his peers to do everything his way. He wouldn't play by the rules. He refused to join games at the park. He stopped playing soccer because he didn't score every time. His need to always win—the game, the sticker for the day, or his teacher's attention—alienated the other kids, and friendships vanished. So did Freddie's joy.

Friends are important for children. Kids who have them feel good about themselves, are more confident, do better in school, and are more likely to grow into well-adjusted adults. Conversely, solitude can lead to isolation, depression, poor health, and discipline problems. One of the most common reasons for friendship issues is a child's behavior. Bossy, disruptive, or self-centered kids annoy their classmates. It's not fun to play with those who don't share or follow rules or who explode when things don't go their way. Shyness and insecurity can also limit a child's friendship circle—as can being different from others, or changes such as a new class or school. Whatever the cause, friendship issues signal a need for extra support and understanding.[6]

The Nine Tools can help get to the bottom of the problem and open options. Your child's imagination is ready to help; Freddie's certainly was. All we needed to do was ask.

When Freddie came in, he was understandably distraught. He needed a safe place to tell his story and listed the worst things in his life:

- "I don't have any friends in my class."
- "Some friends from last year are mean to me."
- "Kids are getting me in trouble for no reason."
- "People I want to play with are playing with people I don't like."

Enter the Feelings Coach: At the same time, he had little awareness of how his own behaviors affected others and burst out crying if someone criticized or corrected him. He was one of those kids who didn't understand the nuances of emotions and needed them broken down. His parents called me his "Feelings Coach."

Consider Some Basic Emotions: I asked Freddie how he felt when kids picked on him. "Awful," he said. I offered, "Awful sad, awful mad, or awful hurt?" so he could zero in on exactly how he felt. "Awful sad." Then I asked him to imagine how he'd like the kids to treat him and how he'd like to feel around them. His answer, again, was vague: "Nice." I gave alternatives: "Nice happy, nice excited, or nice calm?" He picked "happy and excited" and was able to find an image for the feeling: the cheers when his soccer team scored a goal. It was a simple, but significant, step. Now we needed to figure out how he could reach *his* goal.

No Put-Downs: We considered whether Freddie's present behavior would get him to "happy and excited" around his friends. I asked if calling people nasty names would make them be nice to him, or if kind words might work better. Given a clear choice, Freddie chose kind words. He visualized having a pleasant conversation with a classmate, then inviting him to play dodgeball and enjoying himself.

QUICK TIP!   Anyone Can Be a Misfit

Most kids have some trait that inspires teasing—an uncommon name, flaming red hair, a lisp. Perhaps they're extra short or smart or have unusual interests. Other kids, who haven't yet developed a good sense of self, may pick on these differences to boost their ego. But sometimes a child's own behavior ostracizes him. Listen carefully to complaints. Sometimes there is more to the story.

Dog . . . a Boy's Best Friend: Freddie's Animal Friend was his own bulldog, Puggs. I suggested she might bring him a Gift to shed light on why some kids wouldn't play with him. He envisioned a hi-tech lime sphere with a special button that opened it, like a round laptop computer. I asked if anyone from school might send him an email, and indeed, he received a message from a classmate: "I don't want to play with you, you don't play fair!" Whoa—that stung! I recommended he press the button again and see what happened. This time a video popped up from a boy whose feelings got hurt when Freddie teased him. I could see that Freddie felt sorry, so I asked him what happened in those moments. "Sometimes I get so mad at my friends if they don't do what I want," he admitted. "I feel like a tornado." It was a big realization for a little boy.

Clearer Weather Ahead: I gently wondered what it might be like to play with an angry tornado. Freddie agreed that it probably wouldn't be fun. I asked what else his round laptop could show him, and the next touch of the button turned the tide. Freddie pictured a new version of himself: a boy who hadn't made many friends *yet*, but was willing to try and play more calmly. As Freddie resolved to be kinder, we asked for a Gift to help him remember. Puggs gave him a silver medallion to wear. "When you blow on the star, it gives you power to speak nicely," he explained. "I'll keep it in my backpack for school."

Who Else to Approach? Freddie was so pleased with Puggs's Gift that he was open to playing another animal game. I asked him if he could be any animal, what would it be? He stuck with Bulldog, because he'd known Puggs all his life and she was such a loyal friend. I suggested inviting in Animal Friends who reminded him of different classmates. Maybe some would like to befriend his Bulldog. Freddie considered Evan, but he was like a sly snake; that wouldn't do. Michael was a big bouncing puppy, though; surely he'd like another canine companion. And Ricardo had skinny bird legs. Dogs loved to chase birds, so Ricardo made the cut. Freddie continued until he had a list of possible new friends. He returned to school determined to approach these boys and take a chance on some others.

QUICK TIP!   List of Friends

Imagining and making a list of friends is a handy skill. When one pal can't play—whether she's unavailable or just doesn't want to—other choices exist. Your child can remember this on the playground and in planning after-school playdates.

These simple tools changed Freddie's world. Before we knew it, he made another list. Instead of the worst things in his life, he named the best. The first entry: "Making new friends."

HOW-TO FOR YOU

Freddie learned that when you're nice to others, they are kinder to you. Hopefully these ideas can help your child go from friendless to friendly.

Be a Caring Coach

Make sure you're on the same team, even when your child seems to be wrong. It's easy to want to correct your child when you see things so clearly from an adult perspective. But this is not about blame; it's about creating a new beginning. Stay out of the right/wrong discussion; it will only cause power struggles. Instead, let your child know you believe she can make friends. When she feels you on her side, she'll be more open to imagination suggestions—and change.

Imagine Simplicity

Invite her to share her friend situation with you; then ask her to imagine how she'd like it to be. Depending on her age, guide her with simple or sophisticated emotional language. Encourage her to draw present and future possibilities.

Call on Man's Best Friend

Animal assistance—from a dog, cat, jaguar, or ladybug—can provide wise advice and fun Gifts that teach her to create better friendships.

Consider Different Scenarios

Discuss how to make amends with problem friends or reach out to new ones. Role-play together or write a practice script. How would she like her "friendship show" to go?

Reframe the Games

When a child is too competitive, others tire of playing with her. As your child hones her friendship skills through imagery, promote cooperation by changing focus. Asking "Who came in first?" or "What was the score?" inadvertently fuels competition. Instead, inquire whether she had fun, or if the team worked well together. You don't have to ignore who won; just don't make it top priority; she'll learn that games can be about more than winning.

The Final Frontier

Living Lovingly with Parents

An only child, eleven-year-old Grace had always been tough to handle, but in the last two years, everything had become a struggle. Grace wanted more freedom; Mom needed to keep a watchful eye.

Grace thought Mom was overbearing; Mom found Grace inconsiderate. Her parents were braced for trouble at fifteen, even thirteen, but the tween years—nine to eleven—had become a fast-forward to early adolescence. They didn't know what to do. Explosions erupted constantly. Like the day they were shopping at the mall. Grace walked ahead, impatient with her mother's slow pace. Mom felt insulted and also concerned for Grace's safety. She lost her cool and yelled in public. Grace was mortified and angry. Their once close relationship was in tatters. Finally, the family came to me.

Parents often complain about their kids' horrible behavior. They are relieved but dumbfounded to discover that their demon can be an angel with others. "Why don't I ever see that kid?" they ask. If this sounds familiar, take heart. Your child's awful behavior at home is a sign of comfort, of trust in your love and consistency. He knows he can dish out the worst, warts and all, and you won't abandon him. You might chastise, punish, or yell, but you won't stop being his parents. Remember, it's not only teenagers who struggle with uncomfortable issues of identity and changing boundaries. Each stage of development can make a child question who he is and how much freedom he can handle. There's not much difference between the toddler's insistent "Me do it!" and tween rebellion except, of course, the stakes are higher.

Invite your child's imagination into the conversation; it can give you a gentle way to clear the air and validate the deepest part of him as you open communication channels.

When I met Grace, I was struck by her sophistication. She certainly sounded like a teen, although that was still years away. I told her I didn't have answers for her, but she did. If she was open, I could point the way. She agreed. We went over slow breathing as a way to access her internal wisdom. Then, because she caught on quickly, I suggested she check for Animal Friends: "Maybe they can show us what's going on."

Pictures Worth More Than Words: Grace didn't recognize how her behavior affected others. But when Randy Raccoon and Jake Jaguar appeared, volunteering videos of her conduct at home, she described what she saw. First there was a "mean" video where she screamed at her family; then there was a "nice" one where she got along with everyone. I had her imagine stepping into the action and asked her not only how she felt in each scene, but also how she wanted to feel. She preferred staying pleasant and agreeable. With this intention, we were on our way.

Heart Wisdom Is Wonderful: Next, she consulted her Heart. "How can I resolve my conflicts with Mom?" she asked. Her Heart surprised her. "Speak to her," it said. "Understand her point of view, and go from there." Grace was flabbergasted. How could understanding *Mom's* point of view solve this? Heart's wise answer: "When you do, she'll understand yours."

Grace still didn't get it. "Pretend you are her," her Heart continued. "Imagine why she may have done what she did." This was a fun suggestion, given that Grace loved acting. But something still troubled her. "Why can't I forgive her?" Heart thought for a while then said, "You know you love her, but you don't know if what she did shows that she loves you." Grace sighed. It was true, and it felt good to admit it. She softened immediately.

QUICK TIP! **When Kids Surprise Themselves**

No one knows what will surface from your child's imagination—not even him. It's wiser and more truthful than his hurts and worries. Just give him room to listen and discover the power of his own wisdom.

Mirrors and Floating Cloth Offer Solutions: Now that Grace understood her reactions, what could she do about them? I invited her to ask for another image. A mirror showed two hands—hers and her mother's—holding each other. There was a peace sign above them. When she asked about the meaning, she heard, "Work toward peace and friendship. Think positively." What could she do about residual anger? Another picture appeared: a floating green and white checked cloth. It turned bad thoughts into good ones whenever she wiped her forehead on it. Now she felt comfortable about going home and apologizing, and she resolved to be more aware of her part in arguments.

Dad Dominates: Grace's relationship with Mom started improving, but then she began resenting Dad's long work hours. When he was home, he seemed to pick on her for "little things," such as a messy room or too much TV. She felt she could never please him.

Write for Release: Grace couldn't picture how she wanted their relationship to be, so I encouraged her to keep a private diary where she could express her daddy woes. We started in my office, and she had a long list. She felt impatient, cranky, irritated, frustrated, unloved, and overwhelmed. I hoped she could visualize letting go of these intense feelings as she wrote them out. It helped, but there was more. She focused on Balloon Breathing and remembered her Heart's wisdom: see their point of view. From that place, she started to imagine letting love clear her hurts, one at a time.

The Other Hand Holds Insight: Since Grace seemed more willing to understand her parents' side, I thought nondominant writing might let her explore her part. Her "other" hand gave Grace some wise words about improving her situation with Dad.

A Conversation with Grace's Other Hand

DH: How can I keep myself from being rude to Dad?

ND: Keep your mean complaints in your journal.

DH: How can Dad and I live together and bring out our love for each other?

ND: Tell him your true feelings. Be persistent. Don't let his attitude get in the way.

DH: How can I be persistent and not be offensive or make him angry?

ND: Don't tell him his problems—tell him yours.

Vacation Tests the Tide: The situation had been improving until the prospect of a family vacation put Grace to the test. Car trips were hard; during long hours in a small space with no means of escape, views and personalities slammed into each other, and friction festered. In the past, she had screamed at her parents and dissolved into tears. She wanted to keep peace this time but didn't know how. She calmed herself by breathing deeply, closed her eyes, and called in Animal Friends.

Four for the Price of One: Raccoon and Jaguar showed up again with Otter and Koala in tow. They came bearing Gifts and inspiration. Raccoon suggested taking her camera and "art stuff" to scrapbook the family's adventures. Otter recommended that she help with packing and unpacking; Mom would appreciate it. Exasperated, Koala said, "Just have a good time! Don't whine about what you don't want to do." Then she softened. "Enjoy nature, use your time wisely, and let it be fun." Jaguar agreed. "Be nice to everybody, and they will be nice to you." She followed their advice and consulted with them on the trip as needed; it was a great success.

Grace reconnected with the love she felt for her parents—and theirs for her. By practicing the Nine Tools, they also set themselves up for clear communications during adolescence and for life beyond that.

HOW-TO FOR YOU

If you and your tween are struggling to get along, your family will appreciate following Grace's lead.

✴ Listen with an Open Heart

Encourage your child to share his complaints about you. Tell him there will be no recriminations for what he says— what's important is honesty. Set a reasonable time for these talks—hours may be too long, ten minutes too short. Let him know you care about his feelings, and no matter how impossible the situation seems, you can work it out. Don't take his words personally. Instead, listen for the hurt or need behind them. "You never listen to me," is less a statement of fact than a plea for more connection. Nor do you have to give in to every request; just being heard and understood can release resentment. Imagine the relationship you both really want; it's an important first step.

✴ Balance with Good Thoughts

Build trust by telling your child something you appreciate about him daily. Use informal family dinners to share what each of you likes or is grateful for in the other. After a while, kindness will become a habit.

✴ Keep Up with Imagination Technology

If your child is besotted with new technology, use its language to engage your child's imagination when you're trying to communicate better. It puts you in his world. Is TV passé? Maybe he can watch an imaginary iPhone video.

Over email? Go straight to text messaging. Use whatever's "hot" to imagine win-win scenes and scripts that create a loving connection for both of you.

⚏ Connect to the Heart

If you've been encouraging your child to check in daily with his Heart, it will be easy to ask Heart wisdom to shed light on parent-child relations. If not, now is the time to start.

⚏ Write When Talk Doesn't Work

If you have trouble talking to each other, writing can help. Jot down your feelings, thoughts, hopes, and desires for a better relationship. Use your imaginations; along with your Hearts, they are the source of what you'd both like to create. Young kids can dictate; older ones can try the power of their nondominant hand. Exchange notes, thanking each other, and accept whatever is written. It may make initiating a conversation easier.

Connecting from the Heart
An Imagery for Friends and Family

This guided journey can create a heart-centered, loving family atmosphere that meets everyone's needs. If the entire family is participating, you might record the script so you can all share the experience at once and then gather everyone into a circle, facing each other.

We're going to take a vacation from everyday life. Sit in a comfortable position. As you focus on your Balloon Breathing, imagine a favorite place or time when you were happy and peaceful. Get a clear picture of yourself there. What does it look like? Sound like? Smell and feel like? If nothing comes, it's okay to make up something as long as it's soothing.

One of your Guides—an Animal Friend or Wizard carrying a special wand—comes to create a protection circle around you. Decide how big the circle is. Once it's finished, it glows. You are safe inside.

Imagine inviting your family to sit in a circle, inside your protection circle. Trust that anyone who enters loves and accepts you just the way you are. First consider the people you live with—Mom or Dad, your brothers or sisters. Perhaps you'll include your grandparents, or aunts, uncles, and cousins. As each respectfully enters the circle, they take a seat facing you, and each other. Now ask friends to join you. Picture them, one by one. They come, delighted to be part of your extended family.

As you breathe, slowly and deeply, the feelings of love inside you grow stronger. Let go of any squabbles. This is a place to remember you are connected to each other by the love in your Hearts.

Once everyone is settled, imagine the good feelings you have for each person. One by one, focus on your love for them. If you were to send love from your Heart to the person in front of you, on a beam of light or sound, what would it look or feel like? Do you get an image? A color? Maybe you hear music. Whatever you choose is fine. Now send them this love. Imagine receiving their love in return . . . times ten! What is *that* like? How do you feel? Allow their love to completely fill your Heart. It can grow so big that it sends and receives love from everyone. There is always enough to share, and always room for more.

Imagine sending love in any form you wish to another person. Then picture it traveling around your circle and being graciously received. Give yourself permission to absorb their returning love. Take your time. Do this for whoever is with you—your family, your friends, anyone who shows up.

Wow! You have created something magical and unique. What does the center of your circle look like now? Take a few moments to enjoy sharing all this love among you. Imagine each person saying something wonderful to you . . . something you've always wanted to hear. Notice what warm wishes you want to return to them.

You will remember and spread these good feelings as you go about your everyday life. And you can come back to this special circle anytime you like. Now listen as each person says a kind good-bye and quietly leaves the circle. When you are ready, slowly return, bringing all you have learned, all you have felt, into your Heart.

Keep your deep Heart connection with your family and friends. You might like to share, draw, or write some of the images you experienced as a way to remember them.

Afterword

Using the Tools for a Lifetime

★ "Our son is now a delightful, straight A student. He is organized, self-motivated, and self-assured, thanks in no small part to the tools he learned from you. Thank you ever so much!"

"Your Tools have certainly made a difference in our daughter's life. You have helped shape a wonderful young person, who truly believes in herself."

"We are most grateful for all the life lessons we learned as a family because of you."

These are just a few of the notes I've received from parents over the years. They are living testaments to the power of the imagination to change lives. The Nine Tools are more than quick-fix intervention strategies; they are Tools for Life, critical techniques for dealing with whatever challenges your child encounters, at five years old or fifty. These foundation skills will help him develop and maintain self-awareness, self-control, and self-confidence. As you continue to apply and adapt these Tools, you will create a foundation for transforming stress and anxiety into joy and success. You will also create a rich legacy that each child can pass on to his or her own children someday.

Like the kids I meet, my dreams are big. I dream of a world in which real tools for healing and growth are available—and accessible—to every budding Self. I envision a generation of young people who have the imagination and skills to create profound and lasting change. I believe in a future that has a future. The kids themselves prove that it's possible. Consider eight-year-old Bryce, who traveled far in his imagination to a place whose nightly fireworks spelled out "World Peace." He received one Gift: "A little power that gave my Heart the energy to tell the world how I feel about fighting; it changed the world in ten days." And ten-year-old Nancy, who journeyed to many planets to bring special Gifts back to ours—a whole shipload of loving Hearts! When she released them, they spread to every person on Earth, "and they all started to act like people from the Happy Planet!" With visions like these, surely our world can transform. To quote Olympic swimmer Michael Phelps, winner of an "impossible" eight gold medals in 2008, "With so many people saying it couldn't be done, all it took was a little imagination."[1]

What does your child imagine? Let's help make it so.

NOTE FOR PROFESSIONALS

Parents are not the only adults who shape a child's world. Teachers, doctors, nurses, counselors, and therapists have daily opportunities to influence children in positive and lasting ways. The principles of *The Power of Your Child's Imagination* can easily be incorporated into your work as educational and healthcare professionals.

Teachers: Imagination work is a wonderful addition to any classroom. My own journey with imagery began in the schools, and I have trained thousand of educators in these methods. By adapting the Nine Tools to your class, you can help your students develop and maximize their learning potential and friendship skills. One fifth-grade teacher noticed a significant change in student interactions after one semester of "relaxation and imagery." They were kinder and more considerate of one another, and there was less anger and fighting. Wouldn't that be a great change in your class?

Introduce these "imagination exercises" by teaching one Tool a week or one a month. Have the kids sit at their desks or in a circle on the floor; you can even have them lie down if you have space. Read aloud the script for each new Tool or, later on, the imageries at the end of each chapter. Transition times are perfect for this kind of work: after the morning bell, after recess or lunch, or as a gentle way to end the day. Feel free to adapt my imageries, or design your own, to fit specific subjects. Who knows what magic may show up for class!

Pediatricians and nurses: Pediatricians constantly refer their patients to me for help soothing headaches, tummy pains, or anxiety. Yet many of the Tools can be adapted for your office. In just a few minutes, you can engage young patients in imagery techniques that will improve compliance, mood, and even physical health. The Balloon Breath is the quickest way for a child to create inner calm. It takes less than three minutes to explain and another minute to practice. A nervous child can also close his eyes and imagine a Special Place before a required vaccination; the comforting image may distract him from the impending shot. You can teach Color treatment for reducing pain. One pediatric gastroenterologist uses my audiotape with his own son. "I have also recommended it to about 200 of my patients with headaches, abdominal pain, anxiety, diabetes," he wrote. Now you can apply the Tools to your patients. This book is full of ideas. Please use them.

Therapists: Whenever I lecture on the healing power of children's imagination, I watch excitement ignite in psychologists' eyes; it's the same reaction I had so long ago. One therapist at a conference even cornered me with a request: "Please, can you tell me exactly what you do, step by step?" This book does just that. The Nine Tools are easily incorporated into your private practice as a brief cognitive therapy model or for added insight in a longer-term dynamic approach. Whether you work with individuals or groups, imagination is a profound therapeutic tool. Reread the various chapters, and notice which clients come to mind. And, of course, feel free to adapt the imageries to your theoretical orientation, your patient population, and your own personality.

Please Stay in Touch

Imagination work is a dynamic and evolving process. Please email me with your questions, success stories, ideas, and experiences as you continue to make these Tools your own. And log on to my website, www.ImageryForKids.com, to subscribe to my free e-newsletter, or to find out about new articles, upcoming events, and my latest CDs, including *The Power of Your Child's Imagination*, a companion recording of the scripts found in this book.

I look forward to connecting with you all.

Contact Dr. Charlotte at
DrReznick@ImageryForKids.com

ENDNOTES

Introduction. The Power of a Child's Imagination

1 Geoffrey Cowley, "Our Bodies, Our Fears," *Newsweek* (February 24, 2003): 42–50; National Sleep Foundation, *Sleep in America Poll* (2004); William R. Beardslee, MD, and Stuart Goldman, MD, "Kids and Depression: Living Beyond Sadness," *Newsweek* (September 22, 2003): 70; Claudia Kalb, "Troubled Souls," *Newsweek* (September 22, 2003): 68–70.

2 Greenberg-Lake Analysis Group Inc., *Shortchanging Girls; Shortchanging America* (Washington, DC: American Association of University Women, 1991).

3 Jean M. Twenge, PhD, *Generation Me: Why Today's Young Americans Are More Confident, Assertive, Entitled—and More Miserable Than Ever Before* (New York: Free Press, 2006).

4 California Task Force on Self-Esteem and Personal and Social Responsibility, *Toward a State of Esteem* (Sacramento: Bureau of Publications, State Department of Education, 1990).

5 Reuters Health, "Mental Exercise Improves Stroke Outcomes," *Medline Plus* (April 3, 2007); V. Menzies, A. G. Taylor, and C. Bourguignon, "Effects of Guided Imagery on Outcomes of Pain, Functional Status, and Self-Efficacy in Persons Diagnosed with Fibromyalgia," *Journal of Alternative Complementary Medicine* (January–February 2006): 23–30; M. Driediger, C. Hall, and N. Callow, "Imagery Use by Injured Athletes: A Qualitative Analysis," *Journal of Sports Science* (March 2006): 261–71.

6 T. M. Ball, D. E. Shapiro, C. J. Monheim, and J. A. Weydert, "A Pilot Study of the Use of Guided Imagery for the Treatment of Recurrent Abdominal Pain in Children," *Clinical Pediatrics* (July–August 2003): 527–32; B. Hewson-Bower and P. D. Drummond, "Psychological Treatment

for Recurrent Symptoms of Colds and Flu in Children," *Journal of Psychosomatic Research* (July 2001): 369–77; S. A. Lambert, "The Effects of Hypnosis/Guided Imagery on the Postoperative Course of Children," *Journal of Developmental and Behavior in Pediatrics* (October 1996): 307–10; R. D. Anbar, "Self-Hypnosis for Management of Chronic Dyspnea in Pediatric Patients," *Pediatrics* 107, no. 2 (2001): 21–28; R.E.S. Feierstein, "The Use of Guided Imagery to Increase Attention and Academic Achievement in Children with Attention Deficit," *Dissertation Abstracts, The Fielding Institute* (1991): 331; K. Olness and D. P. Kohen, *Hypnosis and Hypnotherapy with Children*, 3rd ed. (New York: Guilford Press, 1996).

7 Paradise Unified School District. Personal communication with author, California Association of School Psychologists Annual Conference (1981).

Chapter 2. How to Get from Here to There

1 Herbert Benson, MD, and Miriam Z. Klipper, *The Relaxation Response*, rev. ed. (New York: HarperCollins, 2000); Jon Kabat-Zinn, PhD, *Full Catastrophe Living: Using the Wisdom of Your Body and Mind to Face Stress, Pain, and Illness* (New York: Bantam Doubleday Dell, 1990); Andrew Weil, MD, *8 Weeks to Optimum Health: A Proven Program for Taking Full Advantage of Your Body's Natural Healing Power*, rev. ed. (New York: Knopf, 2006); Deepak Chopra, MD, and David Simon, MD, *The Seven Spiritual Laws of Yoga: A Practical Guide to Healing Body, Mind, and Spirit* (New York: John Wiley and Sons, 2004); Wikipedia, http://en.wikipedia.org/wiki/hypnosis.

2 Thanks to the meditations learned at the Chee Chung Center in Los Angeles, California.

3 Michael Harner, *The Way of the Shaman*, 10th anniversary ed. (New York: Harper One, 1990).

4 Candace B. Pert, PhD, *Molecules of Emotion: The Science Behind Mind-Body Medicine* (New York: Scribner, 1997).

5 Doc Childre and Howard Martin, *The HeartMath Solution* (New York: HarperCollins, 1999).

6 Claire Sylvia, *A Change of Heart* (New York: Warner Books, 1997); Paul Pearsall, PhD, *The Heart's Code: Tapping the Wisdom and Power of Our Heart Energy* (New York: Broadway Books, 1999); Paul Pearsall, Gary E.R. Schwartz, and Linda G.S. Russek, "Changes in Heart Transplant

Recipients That Parallel the Personalities of Their Donors," *Journal of Near-Death Studies* 20, no. 3 (March 2002): 191–206.

7 Lisa Sloan, PhD, adjunct professor, at Pacifica Graduate Institute, CA. Personal communication with the author.

8 Jeanne Achterberg, PhD, Karin Cooke, BS, RN, Todd Richards, PhD, Leanna J. Standish, ND, PhD, Leila Kozak, MS, and James Lake, MD, "Evidence for Correlations Between Distant Intentionality and Brain Function in Recipients: A Functional Magnetic Resonance Imaging Analysis," *The Journal of Alternative and Complementary Medicine* 11, no. 6 (2005): 965–71. Acknowledgment to the pioneering work using touch of Viola Brody. Viola A. Brody, *Dialogue of Touch: Developmental Play Therapy* (Lanham, MD: Jason Aronson, 1997).

Chapter 3. The Benefits of Artistic Expression

1 American Music Therapy Association, "Frequently Asked Questions About Music Therapy," www.musictherapy.org/faqs.html.

2 Denise Washington, "Does Classical Music Make Babies Smarter?" *BBC News Magazine* (May 19, 2005), http://news.bbc.co.uk/1/hi/magazine/4558507.stm.

3 Don Campbell, "The Mozart Effect Resource Center," www.mozarteffect .com.

4 Linda Weaver Clarke, "Music Soothes the Soul" (May 15, 2006), www .americanchronicle.com/articles/9597; Don Campbell, "How Music Affects Your Child's Brain," http://parenting.ivillage.com/baby/bdevelopment/ 0,,6wk0,00.html.

5 "Symphony News" (January–February 1999), *Music: Food for the Brain*, www.peterperret.com/bolton.html.

6 Rollin McCraty, PhD, Bob Barros-Choplin, PhD, Mike Atkinson, and Dana Tomasino, BA, "The Effects of Different Types of Music on Mood, Tension, and Mental Clarity," *Alternative Therapies in Health and Medicine* 4, no. 1 (1998): 75–84, www.heartmath.org/index2.php?option=com_ content&task=view&id=100&itemid.

7 Don Campbell, *The Mozart Effect: Tapping the Power of Music to Heal the Body, Strengthen the Mind, and Unlock the Creative Spirit* (New York: Harper, 2001).

8 Rebecca Lee, "The Moozart Effect" (May 12, 2007), ABC News, http:// abcnews.go.com/print?id=3213324.

9 Marianne Szegedy-Maszak, "The Art of Healing," *US News & World Report* (2007), www.usnews.com/usnews/9_11/articles/911psych.htm. Acknowledgment to the pioneering work of Joyce Mills in the use of Artistic Metaphor. Joyce C. Mills, Richard J. Crowley, and Margeret O. Ryan, *Therapeutic Metaphors for Children and the Child Within* (New York: Routledge, 1986).

10 James W. Pennebaker, PhD, *Writing to Heal: A Guided Journal for Recovery from Trauma and Emotional Upheaval* (Oakland, CA: New Harbinger, 2004).

11 Lucia Capacchione, *The Picture of Health: Healing Your Life with Art* (Santa Monica, CA: Hay House, 1990).

12 Julia Cameron, *The Artist's Way* (New York: Jeremy P. Tarcher, 1992).

13 "One Year of Writing and Healing: What About the Research on Writing and Falling Apart," www.oneyearofwritingandhealing.com/one_year_writing_and_heal/research/index.html.

14 Lucia Capacchione, *The Power of Your Other Hand: A Course in Channeling the Inner Wisdom of Your Right Brain*, rev. ed. (Franklin Lakes, NJ: New Page Books, 2001); Cat Sanders, "The Power of Your Other Hand: An Interview with Lucia Capacchione," www.drcat.org/articles_interviews/html/lucia.html.

Chapter 5. Everyone Deserves to Be Happy

1 R. W. Robins, K. Trzensiewski, J. L. Tracy, S. D. Gosling, and J. Potter, "Global Self-Esteem Across the Life Span," *Psychology and Aging* 17, no. 3 (2002): 423–34.

2 California Task Force on Self-Esteem and Personal and Social Responsibility, *Toward a State of Esteem* (Sacramento: Bureau of Publications, State Department of Education, 1990).

3 Masuro Emoto, *Messages from Water* (Tokyo, Japan: Hado Kyoikusha Co. Ltd., 2004); Mauro Emoto, *The Hidden Messages in Water* (Hillsboro, OR: Beyond Words Publishing, 2004); Masuro Emoto, *The True Power of Water* (Hillsboro, OR: Beyond Words Publishing, 2005).

Chapter 6. When Life Is Making Your Kid Sick

1 National Pain Foundation, "Pediatric Pain: Psychological Factors Related to Chronic Pain in Children and Adolescents" (2008).

2 "Understanding Role of Stress in Just About Everything," *Science Daily* (January 11, 2008), www.sciencedaily.com/releases/2008/01/080108152439.htm; "Stress: Win Control Over the Stress in Your Life," Mayo Clinic (September 12, 2006), www.mayoclinic.com/health/stress/sr00001; "Stress: Unhealthy Response to the Pressures of Life," Mayo Clinic, www.thestillpointgroup .com/pdf/stress.pdf; U.S. Department of Health and Human Services, Centers for Disease Control and Prevention, *The Effect of Childhood Stress on Health Across the Life Span* (2008), www.cdc.gov/ncipc/pub-res/pdf/ childhood_stress.pdf.

3 The more serious irritable bowel syndrome (IBS) is considered when chronic pain continues for over a year (if other factors are ruled out).

4 "Pediatric Hypnotherapy: Hypnosis Helping Kids," University of Michigan (November 2008), www.med.umich.edu/1libr/yourchild/hypnosis .htm; "Medical Procedures and Pain: Helping Your Child," University of Michigan (January 2007), www.med.umich.edu/1libr/yourchild/med proc.htm.

5 *Ibid.*

6 University of North Carolina in Chapel Hill, http://childpainsolutions .com/information.html.

7 Thomas Ball, MD, et al., "A Pilot Study of the Use of Guided Imagery for the Treatment of Recurrent Abdominal Pain in Children," *Clinical Pediatrics* 42, no. 6 (2003): 527–32; Ran D. Anbar, "Self-Hypnosis for the Treatment of Functional Abdominal Pain in Childhood," *Clinical Pediatrics* 40, no. 8 (2001): 447–51.

8 "Headaches in Children: Common but Sometimes Serious," Mayo Clinic (March 17, 2007), www.mayoclinic.com/health/headaches/HQ00428.

9 Teri Robert, "Let's Study Kids' Head Pain: Symptoms, Diagnosis, Triggers, and Treatment," http://headaches.about.com/cs/children/a/study_ kids_pain.htm (December 1, 2003).

10 "Tics and School Children," *Child Health Monitor* 3, no. 6 (2002), www .keepkidshealthy.com/schoolage/tics_school_children.html; "Tourette Syndrome," Mayo Clinic (May 8, 2008), http://mayoclinic.com/health/ tourette-syndrome/DS00541; Gerald H. Virgilio, "Is It a Tic or Tourette's," *Postgraduate Medicine* 108, no 5 (2000): 175–82; "Tourette's, Other Tic Disorders Far More Common Than Once Thought," *Science Daily* (November 2, 2001), www.sciencedaily.com/releases/2001/11/011101061136.htm.

11 Karen Olness and Daniel P. Kohen, *Hypnosis and Hypnotherapy with Children* (New York: Guilford Press, 1996).

12 "Hypnotherapy of a Child with Warts," *Journal of Developmental and Behavioral Pediatrics* 9, no. 2 (April 1988): 89–91.

Chapter 7. The Bogeyman and Other Scary Stuff

1 Carl Jung, MD, *The Archetypes and the Collective Unconscious* (New York: Pantheon Books, 1959).

Chapter 8. Bedtime

1 "Children's Sleep Problems: What They Are and How to Deal with Them," www.sleep-aid-tips.com/insomnia-in-child-sleep-aid.html; Peg Dawson, EdD, "Sleep and Sleep Disorders in Children and Adolescents," www.nasponline.org/resources/health_wellness/sleepdisorders_ho.aspx.

2 "The Quest for Rest," *Newsweek*, p. 52 (April 24, 2008); "Why We Sleep," www.sleepforkids.org/html/why.html; Vincent Iannelli, MD, "Insomnia and Children," http://pediatrics.about.com/od/sleep/a/0107_insomnia.htm.

3 Hara Estroff Marano, editor at large of *Psychology Today*, email to Valerie Maxwell, PhD, October 24, 2007.

4 "Why We Sleep," www.sleepforkids.org/html/why.html.

5 "Sleep Practices and Tips for Children," www.sleepforkids.org/html/practices.html; "The Sleep of America's Children," www.sleepforkids.org/html/uskids.html.

6 "Co-sleeping FAQ," www.betterforbabies.com/co-sleeping_faq.html.

7 "Why We Sleep," *Time* (December 20, 2004): 48; "Nightwakings," www.kidzzzsleep.org/handouts/nightwakings.htm.

8 Peg Dawson, EdD, "Sleep and Sleep Disorders in Children and Adolescents," www.nasponline.org/resources/health_wellness/sleepdisorders_ho.aspx; Garret D. Evans and Heidi Liss Radunovich, "Bedwetting," University of Florida, http://edis.ifas.ufl.edu/pdffiles/HE/HE79400.pdf; National Kidney Foundation, www.kidney.org; "Bedwetting (Nocturnal Ernuresis)," www.medicinenet.com/bedwetting/article.htm; American Academy of Pediatrics, "Bedwetting," http://patiented.aap.org/content.aspx?aid=5444.

9 Garret D. Evans and Heidi Liss Radunovich, "Bedwetting," University of Florida, http://edis.ifas.ufl.edu/pdffiles/HE/HE79400.pdf.

10 *Ibid.*

11 *Ibid.*

12 Karen Olness and Daniel P. Kohen, *Hypnosis and Hypnotherapy with Children*, 3rd ed. (New York: Guilford Press, 1996): 136–47; Linda Thomson, PhD, "Hypnosis for Children with Elimination Disorders," *Therapeutic Hypnosis with Children and Adolescents* (Carmarthen, UK: Crown House Publishing, 2007): 387–15.

Chapter 9. Why Does Everyone Keep Leaving?

1 J. William Worden, *Children and Grief: When a Parent Dies* (New York: Guilford Press, 1996); J. William Worden, *Grief Counseling and Grief Therapy: Handbook for the Mental Health Practitioner*, 4th ed. (New York: Springer, 2008).

2 Judith S. Wallerstein and Sandra Blakeslee, *What About the Kids? Raising Your Children Before, During, and After Divorce* (New York: Hyperion, 2004); Judith S. Wallerstein, Julia M. Lewis, and Sandra Blakesee, *The Unexpected Legacy of Divorce: The 25 Year Landmark Study* (New York: Hyperion, 2001); Constance Ahrons, *The Good Divorce* (New York: HarperCollins, 1994); Constance Ahrons, *We're Still Family: What Grown Children Have to Say About Their Parents' Divorce* (New York: Harper-Collins, 2004); E. Mavis Hetherington and John Kelly, *For Better of for Worse: Divorce Reconsidered* (New York: W.W. Norton & Co., 2002).

3 *Ibid.*, Charlotte Reznick, *The Long-Term Effects of Parental Divorce on Adolescent Academic Achievement and Psycho-Social Behavior: A Study of Vulnerable and Resilient Children*, unpublished doctoral dissertation (1985), University of Southern California.

Chapter 10. When Good Kids Do Bad Things . . . To Themselves and Others

1 Richard Niolon, PhD, "Dealing with Anger and Children" (December 1999), www.psychpage.com/family/library/angry.html.

2 Kay Kosak Abrams, PhD, "First Comes Hurt, Then Comes Anger and Aggression," *Washington Parent Magazine* (January 2003), www.kayabrams.com/articles/first_comes_hurt.htm.

3 Joshua Mandel, PsyD, Daphne Anshel, PhD, and Staff of NYU Child Study

Center, "Anger: Helping Children Cope with This Complex Emotion," *The Parent Letter* 2, no. 7 (March 2004).

4 *Ibid.*

5 Charles Flatter, James M. Herzog, Phyllis Tyson, and Katherine Ross, Sesame Street Parents, "Anger," www.sesameworkshop.org/parents/advice/article.php?contentid=601&& (accessed July 25, 2008).

Chapter 11. Go For the Gold—Celebrate the Bronze

1 Peg Tyre, "The New First Grade: Too Much Too Soon?" *Newsweek* (September 11, 2006): 34–44.

2 L. Strachan and K. J. Munroe-Chandler, "Using Imagery to Predict Self-Confidence and Anxiety in Young Elite Athletes," *Journal of Imagery Research in Sport and Physical Activity* 1, Article 3 (2006), www.bepress.com/jirspa/vol1/iss1/art3; Ken Kaiserman, *Pressure in Kids' Sports* (November 23, 2005), www.bestsyndication.com/2005/I-Q/kaiserman_ken/112305_kids_sports.htm.

3 Steven Ungerleider, PhD, *Mental Training for Peak Performance: Top Athletes Reveal the Mind Exercises They Use to Excel* (New York: Rodale Books, 2005).

4 Robert Weinberg, *Journal of Imagery Research in Sport and Physical Activity* 3, Issue 1 (2008); "Does Imagery Work? Effects on Performance and Mental Skills," www.bepress.com/jirspa/vol3/iss1/art1; Chris Geier, "Hypnosis Strikes Gold for Amateur, Olympic, and Pro-Athletes" (May 4, 2007), www.hypnosis.edu/articles/sports/performance.

5 Victoria Cunningham, Morty Lefkoe, and Lee Sechrest, "Eliminating Fears: An Intervention That Permanently Eliminates the Fear of Public Speaking." *Clinical Psychology and Psychotherapy* 13 (2006): 183–93.

Chapter 12. Can't We All Just Get Along?

1 Diane McClellan and Lilian G. Katz, "Young Children's Social Development: A Checklist" (1993), http://chiron.valdosta.edu/whuitt/files/social dev.html.

2 Lisa Trei, "New Study Links Reading, Social Skills in Children,"

Stanford Report (February 22, 2006), http://news-service.stanford.edu/news/2006february 22/children-022206.html.

3 Diane McClellan and Lilian G. Katz, "Young Children's Social Development: A Checklist" (1993), http://chiron.valdosta.edu/whuitt/files/socialdev.html; E. R. Christophersen, "Practicing Social Skills with Children," from workshop on Managing Child Behavior Problems at the 2002 American Academy of Pediatrics' National Conference (Boston, October 2002).

4 "My Children Have Trouble Getting Along. How Can I Help Them?" American Academy of Pediatrics, www.aap.org/publiced/br_siblings_rivalry.htm; B. J. Howard, "Helping Siblings Get Along," *Bright Futures in Practice: Mental Health—Vol. II Tool Kit*, M. Jellinek, B. P. Patel, M. C. Froehle, eds. (Arlington, VA: National Center for Education in Maternal and Child Health, 2002), www.brightfutures.org.

5 Jeff Grabmeier, "Siblings Help Children Get Along with Others in Kindergarten," http://researchnews.osu.edu/archive.socskill.htm.

6 "When Children Have Trouble Making Friends," www.fasttrackproject.org/parents.html; Nancy MacNeil, "Help Your Children Get Along with Others," *Bucks County Courier Times*, www1.phillyburbs.com/pb-dyn/news/275=09242007=1412538.html; Robert Hughes Jr., PhD, "Helping Children Get Along with Friends" (May 6, 2008), http://missourifamilies.org/features/divorcearticles/divorcefeature6.htm.

Afterword. Using the Tools for a Lifetime

1 *Los Angeles Times*, "With His 8th Gold Medal, Michael Phelps Is Finally Speechless," August 17, 2008.

INDEX

ABOUT THE AUTHOR

CHARLOTTE REZNICK, PhD, specializes in helping kids develop the emotional skills necessary for a happy and successful life. For over twenty-five years, children and adolescents have been the central focus of her career, her studies, and her imagination. A licensed educational psychologist and associate clinical professor of psychology at UCLA, she has treated children from all walks of life, guiding her clients through the challenges of growing up with her signature style of humor, heart, and imagery. Her secret is simple: Kids learn best when they solve problems for themselves. Rather than give them answers, she teaches kids the tools to find their own truth.

Dr. Reznick is the creator of *Imagery for Kids: Breakthrough for Learning, Creativity, and Empowerment*, a positive coping skills program, and of therapeutic CDs for kids and teens. She is an international expert on the healing power of a child's imagination and a frequent media commentator. Affectionately known as "Dr. Charlotte" by her clients, she maintains a private practice in Los Angeles, California. For information about her speaking engagements, articles, and CDs, visit www.ImageryForKids.com.